PULSE UNVEILED

The Art and Science of Ayurvedic Pulse Reading

PULSE
UNVEILED

The Art and Science of
Ayurvedic Pulse Reading

VICTOR BRIERE, A.D.

Illustrated by Robb Bihun

Published By
The International Institute of Tantric and Vedic Sciences
38921 Sedalia Drive
Gualala, CA
707.225.8844

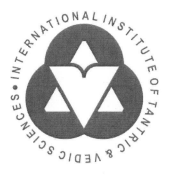

DISCLAIMER

Ayurveda is not considered a medical science by the United States Federal Government nor any State Government. None of the information, images or tables in this book are to be used for medical diagnosis. None of the images in this book were drawn to be or to be understood as medically accurate. They are for visual reference in the context of ayurvedic pulse reading only.

Illustrations by Robb Bihun
All tables created by Victor Briere
Edited by Jennifer Briere and Lisa Wieneke

For more information about Ayurveda, contact:

The International Institute of Tantric and Vedic Sciences
38921 Sedalia Drive
Gualala, CA 95445
707.225.8844
www.iitvsschool.org

THIS BOOK IS DEDICATED TO...

Gurubhai
For seeing the dharma of Ayurveda within me and guiding my heart to a world of greater vision. All without ever reading my pulses...

Bhagat
For having absolute faith in my abilities and providing whatever support I required.

Madison Madden, A.D.
For being my partner in the dharma of Ayurveda, and a living example of a true healer.

Dr. Suhas Kshirsagar and Dr. Manisha Kshirsagar, BAMS
For being my first teachers of the pulse and personally ensuring that my ayurvedic career blossomed.

Dr. Avinash Lele, Dr. Bharati Lele and Dr. Nandan Lele, BAMS
For continuing to teach me the wisdom of Ayurveda from its roots and in its most nuanced and intricate forms.

Dr. Vasant Lad, BAM&S
For unveiling the secrets of the pulse to all those seeking its wisdom.

- And -

Mahan Inder, My Wife
For supporting me more than I'll ever truly know.

Contents

LIST OF IMAGES

LIST OF TABLES

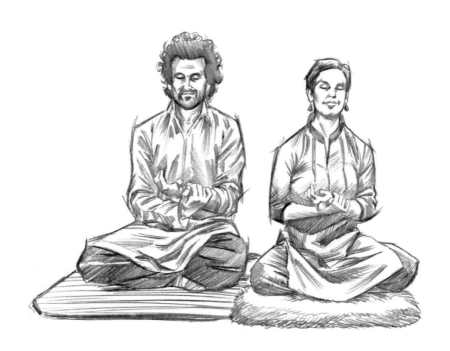

FOREWORD

It gives me great pleasure to write the foreword to this monograph compiled by Victor Briere. Pulse Unveiled is a comprehensive work which will encourage and guide many students to take their first steps into the art and science of pulse reading.

Victor has created a commendable work contained within this praiseworthy monograph. The step by step explanations of pulse reading with beautiful illustrations by Robb Bihun makes it very easy and comfortable for readers to begin *touching* the pulse of the work itself.

Victor demonstrates his devotion and clearly spent a great deal of time and energy in preparing Pulse Unveiled. I am very hopeful that this contribution to the method of pulse reading will serve to inspire the curiosity within the minds of Ayurveda students regarding knowledge of the pulse.

As stated by the author, "It is not simply the pulse reader's task to identify and confirm symptoms. It is the pulse reader's task to truly listen to the body's cry for help and unveil the origin of the imbalance."

Pulse is one of many mediums that can transmit the body's cry for help as well as from where the origin of the imbalance can be ascertained. Ayurveda is a holistic science where all possible angles of the subject are explored to get the complete understanding of that subject. Pulse is one of the eight ways by which one can understand the origin of imbalance. The others are mutra (urine), mala (faeces), jivha (tongue), shabda (sound), sparsha (touch), druk (vision) and akruti (shape/figure/appearance).

It is noteworthy that not much significance was given to pulse reading in classical ayurvedic texts like Charaka, Sushruta and Vagbhata. It was Sharangadhara in 14th Century AD, author of Sharangadhara Samhita who introduced the pulse science in Ayurveda. Thereafter, this knowledge constantly grew and flourished throughout the subsequent period within India. In-fact diagnosis by means of pulse is highly admired by the people of India even in this era of advanced science and technology. However, wise and appropriate use of technology has its own value and importance in the method of diagnosis.

Blessings of a *Guru* (Master)/Apta (Trustworthy source of Knowledge) is pivotal for all students of Ayurveda to be able to download and run an extremely efficient software like pulse reading within his/her system. It is only with constant practice of the beneficial and dispassion towards harmful, purity of the mind, dedication, devotion, determination and discipline that a Guru (Master) bestows his/her blessings over a disciple.

I congratulate the author for the hard work he has taken and wish him all the best for this publication.

Dr. Nandan Avinash Lele
Ayurvedacharya (B.A.M.S)
Tejomay Ayurved, Pune
M.S. INDIA

From the day we entered school for Ayurveda, Victor was determined to become a master pulse reader. Today, in our clinic which sits quaintly on the Northern California coast, each client we receive learns first-hand the profound diagnostic expression of their pulse. Our now students of Ayurveda look forward to learning pulse reading from Victor, knowing of his deep experiential knowledge of this skill that is so valuable and so rare.

It brings me great joy to see this invaluable work added to the Ayurvedic lexicon. It's title, *Pulse Unveiled*, is perfectly suited. It offers a comprehensive introduction to this complex and esoteric subject, and it lays forward a path for those eager to learn the language of ayurvedic pulse reading. It will be a lasting resource to return to again and again.

The knowledge of pulse reading, in my opinion, is one of the most valuable diagnostic skills of a health provider. It is a regular occurrence in our office for the expression in the pulse to accurately proceed a medical diagnosis, and almost certainly to deeply elaborate upon pre-existing medical understandings. The seven-layer pulse methodology provides a vast and precise method to discern the unique expression of health and disease.

While no book can replace the relationship between teacher and disciple, in which Ayurveda is meant to be learned, this work offers a refreshingly straight-forward approach that brings together the biological, spiritual, and historical dimensions of this subject. It honors the traditional heritage of Ayurveda and makes it accessible to the modern student in both the East and West.

I can personally attest to Victor's heartfelt commitment to Ayurveda, to pulse reading, and to the spiritual path that guides it. May this work serve as both a resource and inspiration for those on a similar journey.

Dr. Madison Madden, A.D.
Pacific Coast Ayurveda, Gualala, California

AN INVITATION TO THE ART AND SCIENCE OF PULSE READING

There are legends of pulse readers, some practicing Ayurveda and some practicing Traditional Chinese Medicine, who could perceive the imbalances in someone's body and mind in great detail. They could pin-point diseases which our culture's modern methods of diagnosis miss.

In truth, those masters of the pulse still walk among us. Many have been fortunate enough to meet them. Their pulse. assessments have played a great role in the individual's healing. It is vital to keep this art and science living within our society and living through those who have chosen to discipline themselves to acquiring such a great skill.

This book serves as an instruction manual and guidebook for those who desire to learn the art and science of pulse reading. It is written from an ayurvedic perspective, though many of the techniques are shared with Traditional Chinese Medicine. Reading the book alone will not make one a pulse reader. It is absolutely essential to practice on a daily basis to develop one's nervous system and intuitive capacities in alignment with the art. For that reason, it is exceedingly helpful to find a teacher or teachers of the pulse. Even the teachers of the pulse remain students of the pulse. There is a constant refinement necessary to begin to approach mastery. It is always important to remember that reading an individual's pulse is an intimate affair, and it is vitally important to convey what is felt without bias, with honesty, and with compassion.

In my pursuit of learning the art of pulse reading I have come

1

across a variety of styles within the world of Ayurveda. There is an emphasis on pulse reading in Traditional Chinese Medicine, and a variety of styles underneath its umbrella, and each of those styles also differ from those of Ayurveda. What I have come to learn is that as long as a good portion of the fundamentals remain in-tact, each style presents a form of practice through which the pulse reader can create an intimate relationship. Within that style of practice, the deeper the pulse reader delves, the more refined the pulse reader will become at communicating with the pulse via direct experience.

The pulse is an expression of a unique living being. It is not an artform or science with hard-fast rules or a checklist of movements that guarantee a result just as there is no hard-fast checklist that guarantees a result when sitting down to talk to another human. To engage pulse reading in such a way would limit the pulse reader to his or her rational mind and the subtlety of the pulse reader's experience would be lost. The accuracy of each pulse reading rests on the subtlety, fluidity and intuitive nature of the pulse reader. What is represented in this manual is but one style of pulse reading and is offered to the student as but one structure the student may adopt to assist in her or his growth as a truly focused, nuanced and sophisticated pulse reading master.

The scope of information a student can perceive through the fingertips in incredible. Begin now, without knowing anything else, by placing your fingertips on your wrist as shown on the cover. Take a deep breath and exhale fully. Don't think too much, just feel what is actually there to the best of your ability. This may be your first pulse reading out of thousands. Or, you may already be an experienced pulse reader. Either way, it is a vital exercise to learn how to simply feel an individual's pulses without deducing conclusions.

As you move through this manual you may find certain techniques imperceivable or confusing. If you don't have a pulse teacher to question, simple move on and come back to that section later. Pulse reading is _not_ learned in a linear way. Each pulse reader must unfold his or her perceptive capacities in a more organic, spiralized way. The key point here is not to become discouraged or to try to "figure it out." Simply keep practicing and you will be surprised as to how all of a sudden, you perceive something in the pulse that you could not perceive even the other day.

When you read the pulses of others, especially at the beginning of your practice, ask them for a good deal of feedback and compare what you feel and discern to their experiences of their own bodies. This feedback practice is an art unto itself and will prove invaluable to your learning experience.

While many ayurvedic principles are explained within, this book is not meant to serve as an introduction to Ayurveda. It would be very helpful to the reader to already have an understanding of the basics of Ayurveda such as prakruti, vikruti, and the doshas. In contrast, this book is also not meant to be so advanced that only those extremely seasoned in Ayurveda can apply its contents. A basic understanding of Ayurveda is sufficient to begin practicing. With time and repetition, the practice of the pulse can greatly enrich the student's understanding of the nuances and complexities of Ayurveda. The pulse itself becomes a teacher of ayurveda. One of the great benefits of the art of pulse reading is that it gives the student the direct experience of many ayurvedic truisms, and helps the philosophical aspects come to life.

A large part of this manual is to encourage the student to unlock his or her intuitive capacities while reading the pulse. This does not mean "magically" know what is going on in someone's body. Rather, it means to learn to synthesize the information taken in through the fingertips in a non-rational manner. To train one's system to ascertain extremely subtle messages by quieting the rational mind. In this way, the practice of pulse reading is a meditation and thusly an invitation to practice Yoga. In the study of Ayurveda, you will find that many of the techniques benefit not only the recipient, but the practitioner as well. This attitude towards healing blossoms from the core belief that the pulse reader and the one seeking help, the rogi, are of one spirit.

Now let's begin with the basics…

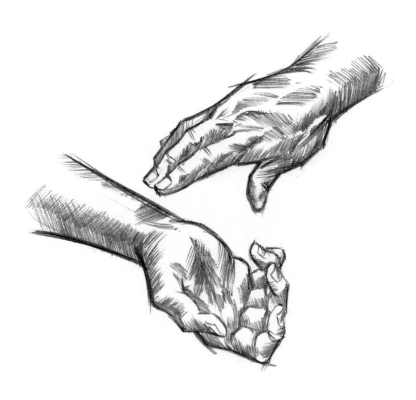

CHAPTER ONE

A PROPER TECHNIQUE

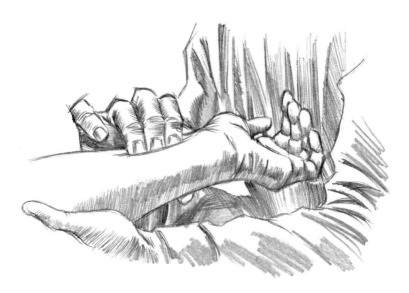

Image 1 - Proper Technique

In Ayurveda the art of pulse reading is named <u>nadi pariksha</u> or <u>nadi vijnana</u> which literally translates to pulse exam or pulse diagnosis. The pulses are typically read on the thumb's side of the wrist. Just below the heel of the palm, on the thumb's side, the pulse reader will feel the tip of the radial tubercle. Place the index finger below this protrusion, towards the heart, and slightly inward. Feel around that area until the radial artery has been identified.

Angushta moola bhage ya dhamani jiva sakshini |
Tat cheshtaya sukham dukham gyanam kayasya panditaha ||

The artery pulsating at the base of the thumb should be specially examined.

5

The perceived movements felt by an expert express a state of happiness or unhappiness within the mind and body.

-Vasav Rajiya

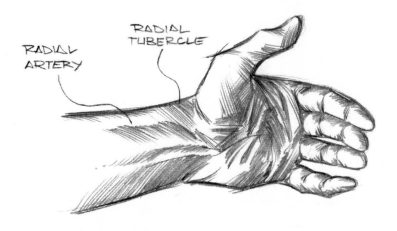

Image 2 - Radial Artery

There are a number of reasons the pulse is most frequently read in this location. Most of them are practical. It is an easily accessible area on the body. The rogi, defined as "the one in distress," does not need to undress. The artery is close to the surface of the skin and can be clearly located. Most importantly, from a healing perspective however, the majority of rogis can remain calm, comfortable and are willing to be touched in this area. As mentioned previously, pulse reading carries a certain level of intimacy between the pulse reader and the rogi. A nervous rogi will present quite different pulses. Although this is important information in and of itself, there is no advantage to creating undue stress or   discomfort when reading the pulse.

Remove the index finger from the radial pulse. Align the index, middle and ring fingers on as even of plane as possible with the pinky lifted, as shown below.

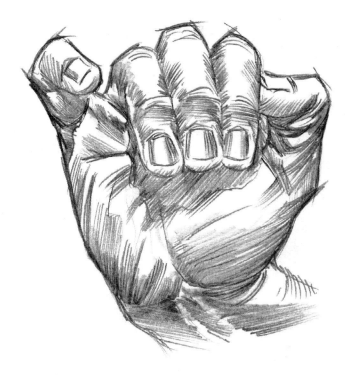

Image 3 - Fingertips on a Single Plane

This is the starting position. It is important that all three fingers touch the radial artery at the same time and on the same plane. The pulses are read with the fingertips and <u>not</u> the pads of the fingers. The fingers should be together, relaxed, either with the sides touching gently or *very* slightly apart.

COMMON MISTAKE

It is very common for beginning pulse readers to break the plane that runs across the three fingertips as the pulse reader delves into the different layers of the pulse. Some of the more advanced techniques require breaking this plane. However, for now, practice keeping this plane intact. The three fingers should move as a single unit. This frequently takes pulse readers quite a bit of practice before it feels natural. When in doubt, simply remove the fingers from the pulse, re-align them, and begin again

The very first impression a pulse reader receives when feeling a rogi's pulse is often one of the most important.

The pinky is lifted as it is not used for pulse assessment. It should not touch the rogi's skin as information carried through the pinky can add distracting sensory inputs. The thumb is underneath the rogi's wrist to support the pulse reader's hand. When reading one's own pulse the thumb need not be under the wrist. It can be off to the side.

The pulse reader will very lightly place three fingers on the radial artery and apply only as much pressure as necessary to begin perceiving the pulse. This is the first layer of the pulse. A pulse will most often be felt under each fingertip. Although, it is not uncommon that the pulse will be absent under the ring finger on the first layer. While this is a sign of imbalance, it is a common one. Unless an imbalance is present, the pulse will be felt under all three fingertips on the first layer.

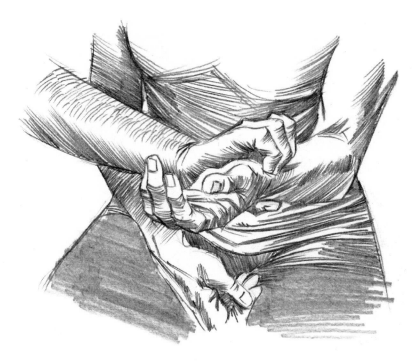

Image 4 - Improper Form

8

IMPROPER FORM

The above image is an example of improper form for two reasons. The first is that the ring finger is closest to the rogi's thumb. The second is that the pulse reader's arm is crossing the entirety of the rogi's body. Overall, the pulse reader is in an awkward position in relation to the rogi and would inappropriately have to break proper posture to achieve the above positioning.

PROPER FORM

There are two schools of thought regarding whether the fingertips can cross the rogi's wrists as shown in in the below image. As can be seen, the fingertips are in the proper position with the index finger closest to the thumb, but instead of reading the rogi's radial artery from the outside of the wrist, the pulse reader's fingers arch across the rogi's wrist to reach the pulse. This is a common occurrence if the pulse reader uses his or her right hand to read the radial artery of the rogi on the right side or vice versa.

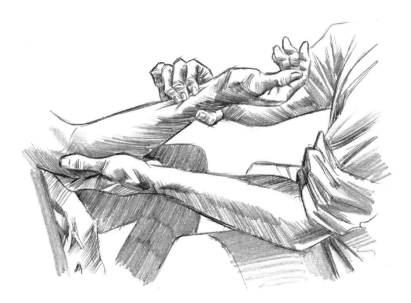

Image 5 - Proper Form for Crossing the Wrist

One school of thought is that the above image does not represent an appropriate way to read the pulse. In other words, the pulse should always be read from the outside of the wrist. In this case, if the pulse reader were to read both of a rogi's wrists, the pulse reader would use his or her right hand to read the rogi's left wrist and her or his left hand to read the rogi's right wrist.

The other school of thought is that it is acceptable to cross the wrist. The image above is one of the proper methods. This style is encouraged for those who prefer to use one hand predominately to read pulses. In this case the pulse reader would use the same hand to read both the rogi's right and left wrists. The student may choose either style so long as proper posture, breathing and finger positioning on the radial artery are honored.

A BRIEF NOTE ON HYGIENE

The pulse reader should have her or his nails trimmed as to avoid digging into the skin of the rogi and leave marks or obstruct the pulse reader's fingertips. The pulse reader's hands should be clean and dry.

POSTURE

Proper posture is crucial to pulse reading. Traditional pulse readings were performed with the pulse reader sitting either cross-legged, in half lotus, or in full lotus. The single most important factor in regard to posture is to maintain an erect spinal column. This can be accomplished sitting in a chair as well, which is how most pulse reading is contemporarily performed.

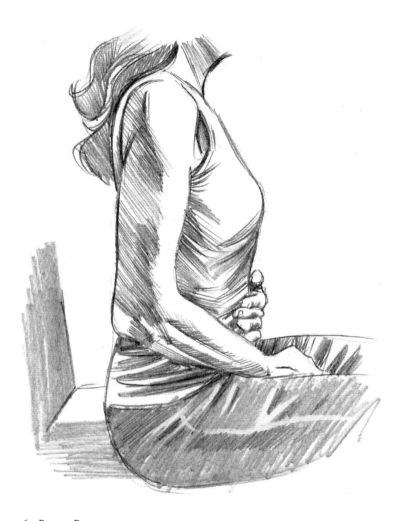

Image 6 - Proper Posture

An erect spine has many benefits. The most crucial component is to allow for the full expansion of the diaphragm which allows the breath to flow freely. If the breath does not flow freely then the pulse reader cannot be fully relaxed.

A tense pulse reader has far more difficulty perceiving the subtle messages of the pulse. A relaxed pulse reader has the opportunity to read pulses via his or her intuition.

An erect spine encourages the flow of cerebral spinal fluid to the brain, amplifying the pulse reader's sensory perception potential.

11

Below is an example of improper posture.

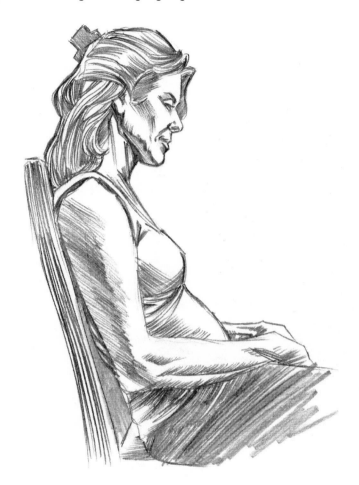

Image 7 - Improper Posture

BREATHING

The importance of breathing properly when reading the pulse, and at all other times, is absolutely foundational to the development of pulse reading. Held within the breath is our consciously accessible ability to dramatically change the functionality of our nervous and sensory systems within a very short period of time.

The quality of the pulse reader's breath is as important, if not more important, than the quality of the pulse reader's fingertips. The pulse reader begins by placing the fingertips on the radial artery, inhaling deeply through the nose and exhaling through the nose. The breath should be long, slow, relaxed, natural and deep while reading the pulses. The abdomen should expand at the beginning of the inhale prior to the expansion of the chest cavity. The abdomen should contract towards the spine during the exhalation. If this is not the case, then practicing a breathing exercise is absolutely essential until this method of breathing becomes second nature.

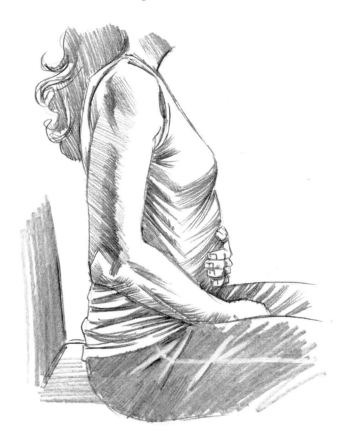

Image 8 - Expanding the Abdomen Upon Inhalation

The practice of pulse reading and the practice of breathing should become synonymous over time. Proper breathing allows the pulse reader to enter his or her parasympathetic nervous system and will dramatically reduce the experience of projecting personal biases onto the information gathered from the rogi's pulse.

Prior to reading a rogi's pulse, the pulse reader should use the breath to ensure that he or she feels centered and grounded. The pulse reader may also use this opportunity to mentally chant a mantra. Repetition of a ritual such as this trains the pulse reader's nervous system to enter a state condusive to pulse reading and creates a calm, attentive, soothing demeanor.

EYES AND VISON

There are a few different methods of holding the eyes that the pulse reader may adopt according to her or his natural inclination. The important underlying factor is that the eyes remain relaxed and soft. The eyes utilize a large portion of attention at any given time. The human body is innately wired to prioritize visual stimulation in many situations. So much information flows into our nervous system through the eyes that visual stimuli can be a source of distraction while reading pulses. Eye strain and subtle eye tension is a common disturbance and has a significant impact on the sensitivities of the other senses.

In Ayurveda, the mind can unite with a particular sense organ at any given moment so that the perceiver can focus on the information being "touched" by that sense organ.

This profound axiom of Ayurveda can be acutely experienced by the student. In Ayurveda, touch is the foundational sense from which all other senses are derived. In this way, the eyes "touch" the object of vision. More importantly for the pulse reader, is the minds ability to unite with a particular sense organ and tune out the information coming in via the others. This allows for a heightened experience of that singular sense. Training the capacity to tune into and intensely focus on one's sense of touch, especially in the fingertips, creates specialized nervous system pathways inside of and unique to the pulse reader. As with meditation, pulse reading is a practice in developing a form of single-pointed focus.

The pulse reader may either close his or her eyes completely, keep the eyes 1/10th open, or keep the eyes open completely as long as they are relaxed.

14

COMMON MISTAKE

Some pulse readers are tempted to look into the rogi's eyes or at the rogi's face while reading pulses. The pulse reader should <u>not</u> do this. Too much information is transferred from the face and eyes for the pulse reader to remain completely focused on the information coming in via the fingertips. Information transferred via faces and eyes has a special impact on the pulse reader's autonomic nervous system and gets automatically processed on both a conscious and a subconscious level.

Practice pulse reading with all three forms of eye posture to see what feels most natural.

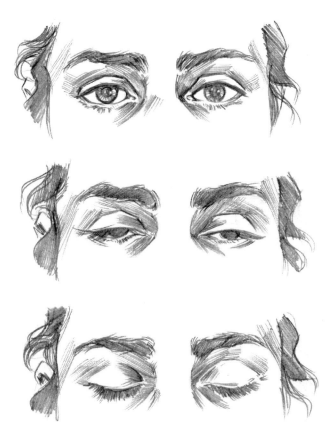

Image 9 - Eye Postures

In the beginning, it is very beneficial to read pulses in a relatively quiet area free from common distractions. When one's ability to focus improves, this becomes less important as the pulse reader's mind is trained to ignore inputs from the other sense organs while reading pulses.

The pulse reader may also request that the rogi close his or her eyes. This helps the rogi draw her or his attention inward and remain focused on the pulse reading as well. When the intention and attention of the pulse reader and the rogi unite, the channels of communication open more completely.

READING A FEMALE'S PULSE VERSUS A MALE'S PULSE

Traditionally a pulse reader will read the male's pulse on the right radial artery and a female's pulse on the left radial artery. The right-side pulse for a male is more expressive of the subtle components of a male anatomy and vice versa for a female. The ayurvedic principle that lies behind this is that generally, the male anatomy is more influenced by the solar channel in the body and the female anatomy is more influenced by the lunar channel. The solar channel, referred to as the pingala, originates on the right side of the body. The lunar channel, referred to as the ida, originates on the left side of the body. The ida and pingala will be explored further in chapter three.

Some styles of pulse reading maintain this practice strictly. Other styles will read both wrists regardless of the gender of the rogi. All of these options will be explored. In general, the student of the pulse can read a male's right-side first and a female's left-side first before switching to the other wrist.

APPROACHING THE ROGI

The way in which the pulse reader approaches the rogi influences both the pulse reader and the rogi. It is an opportunity to either gain or lose trust and thusly impacts the efficacy of the delivery of the information discerned during the pulse reading. Approaching the rogi, orienting the body correctly to the rogi's body, moving gracefully, confidently and kindly, sends a message to the rogi that she or he can relax, especially when the rogi has never experienced a pulse reading before. Jerky, insecure, unprepared movements can engender a sense of suspicion in the rogi.

The pulse reading begins the moment the rogi's wrist is requested, if not before.

Prior to reading the pulse, the pulse reader should request that the rogi remove all watches, wrist bands, wrist jewelry and move the sleeves on both arms up and out of the way. Once the pulse reading begins, this process should not have to be repeated on the opposite wrist, which can break the focus of the pulse reader.

The rogi's wrists should be at approximately the height of the rogi's diaphragm. The rogi's arm should be relaxed, either resting on a stable surface or embraced by the pulse reader's arm.

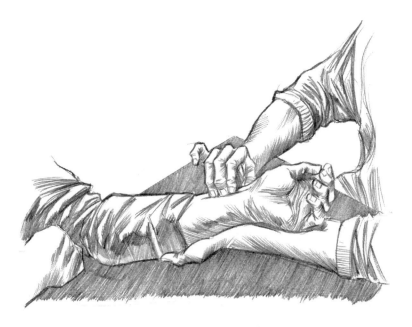

Image 10 - Using a Desk or Table as Support

If the pulse reader feels tension in the rogi's arm then she or he may request the rogi to breath, relax, and if appropriate, encourage the rogi's arm to relax by gently shaking it. The pulse reader should also make sure that the rogi has a relatively erect posture. The rogi should not be slumped or collapsed whenever preventable. Once the proper posture, orientation and relaxation are present, the pulse reader may place his or her fingertips on the radial artery.

TIMING

While seldom possible in a modern clinical setting, the ideal time to read a rogi's pulse is during the hour before sunrise, after the rogi has relieved him or herself of any bowel and urinary urges, and before the rogi engages in the day's variable happenings. It is in this condition that the rogi's pulses most clearly express the underlying state of the body. It is also during this time that the rhythms of the natural world, and those within the pulse reader, support clear intuitive insight.

The pulse reader can make many internal adjustments to the reading to compensate for a rogi's daily activities. For instance, if the pulse reader takes the rogi's pulse just after eating, then kapha will likely be more prominent throughout the pulse. Knowing this, the pulse reader would not unwittingly identify this expression as a systemic kapha aggravation. In general, the pulse reader should not read an individual's pulse just after the individual exercises or becomes highly emotional. In these cases, the pulses temporarily express high levels of pitta and vata that subside after a short time.

COMPLETENESS

A complete pulse reading consists of perceiving information from:

1. All the layers of the pulse, of which there are seven.
2. The qualities present within each layer.
3. The locations of each point of contact on each fingertip.
4. The characteristics of the pulse such as rate, rhythm, gait, force, volume, temperature, and texture
5. The pulse as a whole.

Each of these will be explored in detail in later chapters. The pulse reader is ultimately moving towards a holistic pulse assessment and should not remain fixed on a single or a few details to the disregard of the whole.

As with any practice, the basic techniques create form and structure for deeper experiences within the art. Practice them repeatedly until they are engrained and second nature. It is very common for a pulse reader to "forget" to apply a particular basic technique well into her or his development. This is a good indication of deep-seated resistance within the practitioner, which is in some way related to that technique. Creating a new habit through repetition can help unlock unexpected experiences for the student of the pulse.

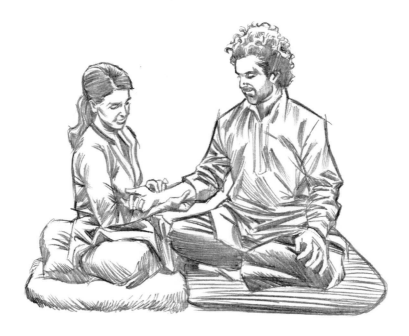

Image 11 - Cross Legged Pulse Reading

CHAPTER TWO

EXPERIENCING QUALITIES
IN THE PULSE

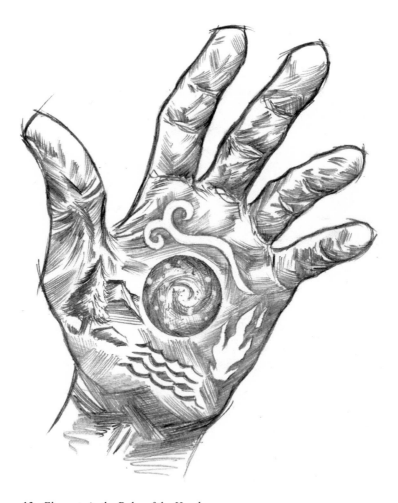

Image 12 - Elements in the Palm of the Hand

Cool, warm, thin, prickly, slippery, light, empty, dispersing, heavy, sticky, plucky, strong, sharp, electric, soft, muted, stunted, hidden, subtle, stable, unstable, steady, unsteady, broad, erratic, dull, explosive, distressed. These are a few examples of qualitative language a pulse reader can use to describe her or his experience when reading the different layers of the pulse.

Strictly speaking, there is no limit to the amount of qualitative words or phrases a pulse reader can use to describe the status and activities within the body as long as the pulse reader's self-talk accurately reflects the truth.

The qualities experienced via the fingertips during a pulse reading are the building blocks of deeper assessment. They suggest activities, or lack thereof, belonging to the three doshas vata, pitta, kapha, subdoshas, tissues (dhatus), sub-tissues (upadhatus), bi-products (malas), and rajas/tamas/sattva (gunas). Each of these will be explained more fully in the chapters pertaining to their relevant layers of the pulse.

THE IDEAL PULSE

Before exploring the varied and nuanced qualities expressed by the pulse, the pulse reader should undertand, in simple terms, what an ideal pulse feels like. This provides a benchmark for all pulse readings.

Suvyakta Nirmala ch eva, swa sthan sthiti eva cha|
Achanchalya Amandatvam sarvasa lakshanam shubham||

An ideal pulse is clearly expressed, not hidden, free of impurities, in its own location, not too brisk and not too slow.

It radiates a feeling of auspicious balance at all levels.

-Vasav Rajiya

This passage is intentionally broad sweeping. The features described will be subject to the individual's prakruti. The passage means to convey a holistic, overall quality that the pulse reader must train

21

him or herself to notice and capture. With practice, the student of the pulse will find him or herself noticing whether a pulse simply feels "sick" or, in the words above, "radiates auspiciousness" prior to diving into the details of each layer

THE BASIC QUALITIES

The most basic qualities every pulse reader should train him or herself to feel clearly are represented below. They come from the classical wisdom of Ayurveda and apply to the body of Ayurveda in general. At first appearance, not all of these qualities seem to apply to the pulse. Such as 'solid' or 'rough'. However, as the pulse reader explores all of the different aspects of pulse reading, the appearance of the qualities becomes quite frequent. Often, they are experienced as lack of their opposites. For example, a pulse that contacts the fingertip abruptly, without gliding across the surface smoothly, will be experienced as rough or 'not smooth' in comparison. A pulse that has a hammering quality as though something is striking the fingertip without conforming fully to the curvature of the fingertip could be experienced as both 'hard' and 'solid,' or, 'not liquid/fluid.'

Each pulse contains a multitude of qualities, intermixed and expressing themselves simultaneously.

THE FUNDAMENTAL TWENTY QUALITIES

HEAVY	LIGHT
SLOW	FAST
COLD	HOT
UNCTUOUS (OILY)	DRY
SMOOTH	ROUGH
SOLID	LIQUID
SOFT	HARD
STATIC	MOBILE
GROSS	SUBTLE
CLOUDY	CLEAR

A student of the pulse sits with proper posture and practices proper breathing. Eyes relaxed, the pulse reader places the fingertips on the first layer of the radial artery. The pulse reader begins to interpret the feelings you experience by the qualities they convey.

The most prominent quality on the first layer of the pulse should be given special notice.

The pulse reader should resist the temptation to jump to conclusions, continue to feel and ask him or herself, "Which qualities are present in a more subtle form or are background to the most prominent quality? Which qualities are absent altogether? Are there any qualities that appear to come and go?" That is a quality in and of itself.

When first starting out, some find it helpful to write down experiences immediately afterwards. It is up to each individual pulse reader as to how helpful this practice is. Most important is repetition over a wide variety of pulses over a wider range of times of day, seasons, ages and life situations.

A pulse reader should read his or her own pulses multiple times each day in a variety of situations to experience first-hand how the qualities change according to different internal and external circumstances.

With repeated practice the pulse reader will become acquainted, and ultimately intimate, with the qualities of the pulse. In time, the pulse reader will develop her or his own self-talk. This inner language will only be relevant to the pulse reader but is an integral part of the development of the skill, and in most students comes naturally.

COMMON MISTAKE

Some pulse readers have a tendency to create elaborate descriptions of the underlying qualities experienced in the pulse. They use complex metaphors and abstract concepts in their own self-talk. This creates an inclination to enmesh the rational mind in the pulse reading process. Remember that these qualities are primal, fundamental building blocks that are readily experienced in nature and not complex philosophical abstractions. Keep self-talk simple, honest, and most importantly, in direct alignment with the actual sensations delivered by the pulse itself.

QUALITIES AND THE ELEMENTS

Ayurvedic assessment, at its heart, is based on the qualities displayed by the primordial elements. The qualities the pulse reader picks up on during a reading correlate to these elements, which then correlate to the three doshas - vata, pitta and kapha. As the rogi's pulse expresses information through the pulse reader's fingertips, these correlations begin to unfold to the pulse reader's intuitive senses. Beginning with the qualities, a pulse reader can experience a rogi's physiological makeup in terms of the elements.

A substance and its qualities, and thus its functions, are inseparable.

This extraordinarily insightful ayurvedic axiom expresses the wisdom by which a pulse reader can confidently make the leap between experiencing qualities and _knowing_, not deducing, that the qualities being experienced represent the basic constituents, described as elements, that make up every portion of the physical form and beyond. These elements are the physical particles by which all forms are created. Later, the pulse reader will also rely on this axiom to assess the function of specific systems, tissues and organs in the body.

THE ELEMENTS AND SOME OF THEIR CORRESPONDING PULSE QUALITIES

ELEMENT	CORRESPONDING QUALITIES
AKASH - ETHER	EMPTY, SPACIOUS, CLEAR, SUBTLE, WITHOUT FORM
VAYU - WIND	MOBILE, SUBTLE, RAPID, THIN, ERRATIC, ROUGH
AGNI - FIRE	HOT, SHARP, PENETRATING, FORCEFUL, CONSTANT, JUMPY
JALA - WATER	SMOOTH, SOFT, SPREADING, COOL, FLOWING, CONNECTIVE
PRITHVI - EARTH	SMOOTH, SOFT, COLD, DENSE, STICKY, CLOUDY, BROAD, SLOW, DEEP

The pulse reader begins to interpret the feelings experienced by the fingertips by the qualities they convey. Without hesitation, the student correlates all of the qualities being conveyed into elemental terms. If there is confusion or doubt the student ignores it and simply transitions his or her self-talk from being focused on qualities into being focused on their corresponding elements. As the student practices this technique and the transition becomes seamless, the student may begin to experience a deeper flow of information. The prominence of one or two elements expressed by the pulse gives the pulse reader definitive information of the physiological makeup of body.

For example, if the pulse reader, while reading the first layer of the pulse, experiences a predominance of the hot, forceful and erratic qualities, then the pulse reader _knows_ that there is a strong presence of agni and vayu in the physiology. The pulse reader will pick up on many qualities while reading a rogi's pulse at any given moment, however, specific qualities will certainly present themselves more prominently than others.

COMMON MISTAKE

Many pulse readers engage in doubt and confusion surrounding what is actually being felt. This in and of itself isn't so much of an issue if it can be dropped. The real issue is that these doubts and confusions tend to encourage the pulse reader to focus on him or herself, which steals the focus away from the pulses. When doubt and confusion arise, simply return the attention to the fingertips and the pulse without hesitation.

QUALITIES AND THE DOSHAS

From the elements arise the doshas. Vata, pitta and kapha. Each dosha is created by the mixture of two elements. Doshas are important to the pulse reader because they perform a wide array of very unique and specific functions in the body. The doshas are in constant relationship with each other at all times. They fall in and out of balance with each other constantly. An individual's health is determined by how well the doshas are harmonizing with each other within a singular, whole system. The balanced, healthy development of the tissues and organs is dependent upon the continued balance of the doshas.

A pulse reader _knows_ which doshas are prominent and how they are acting via the information ascertained from the qualities and the elements.

THE DOSHAS AND THEIR MAKEUP

DOSHA	ELEMENTAL COMPOSITION	FUNDAMENTAL QUALITIES
VATA	AKASH AND VAYU	LIGHT, FAST, DRY, ROUGH, MOBILE, SUBTLE, CLEAR, NEUTRAL IN TEMPERATURE
PITTA	AGNI AND JALA	HOT, LIQUID, SUBTLE, UNCTUOUS, LIGHT
KAPHA	JALA AND PRITHVI	HEAVY, SLOW, COLD, UNCTUOUS, SMOOTH, SOLID, SOFT, STATIC, GROSS, CLOUDY

When reading pulses, transition the self-talk from qualities to elements and then again from elements to doshas. The prominence of one or two elements informs the pulse reader as to the prominence of a specific dosha or doshas. For example, if the pulse reader experiences a prominence of the akash and vayu elements then the pulse reader <u>knows</u> that there is a prominence of vata on the first layer of the pulse.

Here, a level of sophistication is required from the pulse reader. Many of the elements share select qualities and both pitta and kapha share jala in their elemental makeup. If a pulse reader were to experience a prevalent quality that is shared between elements, or a predominance of the jala element, the pulse reader needs to incorporate other information in order to discern which dosha is expressing itself most prominently.

The elements share qualities, and pitta and kapha share an element because there is an underlying similarity in their behavior within nature. In the case of pitta, the flowing quality of jala combined with the penetrating quality of agni gives the pitta dosha its acidic nature. In the case of kapha, the flowing quality of jala combined with the resilient quality of prithvi give the kapha dosha its malleable, clay-like nature. These are two examples of many. Different combinations of qualities give rise to the different functional aspects of each dosha. By becoming intimate with the many permutations and combinations of qualities, elements, and doshas, the pulse reader develops an intuitive sense of the complex functions associated with the myriad of potential combinations.

The intuitive sense need not thumb through innumerable tables and charts to select the appropriate combination of qualities, elements and doshas. There are too many. The pulse reader develops the ability to perceive the most important and relevant information based on perceiving specific patterns in the pulse. Some ayurvedic sages are referred to as acharyas, which means, "pattern perceivers" in acknowledgment of their advanced ability to do just that. Repetitive practice on a variety of different pulses is imperative to sensitizing the pulse reader to an ever-expanding arena of different experiences. When learning pulse reading, qualities, elements and doshas should not truly be considered separate though it can be useful to describe them in such terms. They are different forms and patterns of the same basic materials.

CHAPTER THREE

FUNDAMENTAL CHARACTERISTICS OF THE PULSE

Along with the qualities, all pulses have certain characteristics that provide the pulse reader with valuable information. Every pulse reader should pick up on these characteristics each time she or he reads a pulse. Many of the characteristics will "carry" the qualities that the pulse reader is already familiar with at this point.

1. The pulse rate
2. The rhythm in which the pulse expresses itself
3. The gait of the pulse - the manner in which the pulse travels across the point of contact
4. The amount of force with which the pulse impacts the fingertips
5. The volume of blood that moves through the pulse with each beat
6. The surface temperature of the skin where the pulse is read
7. The texture of the veins/arteries themselves

THE PULSE RATE AND RHYTHM

The pulse rate is how many times the pulse touches the fingertips each minute. The pulse rhythm is the amount of time that passes between each beat. The pulse rate and rhythm will likely remain consistent through all the layers of the pulse. The vata dosha is the only dosha that possesses the quality of movement and plays a large factor in determining the pulse rate and rhythm. Individuals with an abundance of vata activity in their system will have a faster pulse rate of approximately eighty to ninety beats per minute. Individuals with an abundance of pitta activity in their system will have a moderate pulse rate of seventy to eighty beats per minute. Individuals with an abundance of kapha activity in their system will have a slower pulse rate of fifty to sixty beats per minute. All of these pulse rates represent a resting pulse rate. Individuals with very strong circulatory and cardiac function will express a more kapha-like pulse rate.

Contained within the measuring of the pulse rate and rhythm resides a technique that unveils a wellspring of information for the pulse reader. A respiratory sinus arrythmia is the change of heart rate, and thus pulse rate, caused by the inhalation and exhalation of the rogi. The heart rate is largely governed by the strength of the vagus nerve. The vagus nerve persistently signals the heart to keep a specific rate and rhythm by applying what is called the "vagal brake." When the vagal break is suppressed, the heart rate increases. The vagus nerve runs from the brain stem all the way to the reproductive organs right through the diaphragm. The movements of the diaphragm send constant communication to the heart via the vagus nerve.

The connection between the heart, the diaphragm and the breath via the vagus nerve is one of the most profound connections in the body

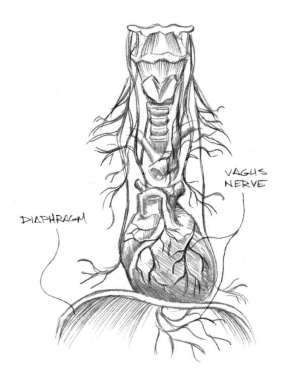

VAGUS
NERVE

DIAPHRAGM

Image 13 - The Vagus Nerve Innervating the Heart and Diaphragm

The pulse reader may ask the rogi to take a deep inhalation. This will suppress the vagal break and the heart rate will increase. Exhalation will relieve the pressure, the vagal brake will re-engage, and the heart rate will decrease. The extent to which a pulse reader experiences an increase in heart rate upon deep inhalation and then the decrease in heart rate upon exhalation, is the extent to which she or he can discern the healthy function of the vagus nerve. Healthy vagus nerve functions suggests that the rogi is able to dwell in the parasympathetic nervous system more readily.

It is in the parasympathetic nervous system that balanced digestion, tissue regeneration, and most healing occurs.

The complete absence of a respiratory sinus arrythmia, or a very weak one, in which the heart rate change is barely perceptible (one or two beats per minute faster or slower) signals the pulse reader that the vagal tone is weak and that the rogi too easily enters the sympathetic nervous system. The sympathetic nervous system governs defensive behavior and physiological functions such as fight, flight, freeze and immobilization responses. Healing and digestive functions are deprioritized when the body is in a sympathetic nervous system response. Spending extended periods of one's life in the sympathetic response is a common causal factor in the development of disease.

If a rogi dwells frequently in the sympathetic nervous system, it can be an indication that the rogi will experience more difficulty in adopting and sustaining the pulse reader's suggestions. Rogis with a weak vagal tone, or rogis that are actively engaged in a defensive mentality have a more difficult time making changes especially those that encourage healing. It is likely that the rogi has become dependent on unhealthy habits to maintain a semblance of safety and control. These habits contribute greatly to the disease pathology and are simultaneously the most difficult for the rogi to willingly give up. The pulse reader can become aware of all of this through understanding the pulse rate.

COMMON MISTAKE

Many pulse readers forget to take the time of day, the current emotional state, and the rogi's immediately prior activity into account when drawing information from the pulse rate. It is very common for a rogi's pulse rate to be higher during mid-day and lower in the early morning and at night. The pulse rate will frequently be higher if the rogi is nervous, anxious or afraid. Sometimes simply being in a clinician's office creates anxiety in the rogi that he or she will not communicate until asked directly. The rogi's immediately prior activity affects the pulse rate significantly. If the rogi was just exercising, eating, arguing, driving, etc., then the pulse rate will reflect this. There is no right or wrong time to take the pulse, as long as these factors are accounted for by the pulse reader.

THE GAIT

The gait of the pulse is the pattern of the pulse's movement across each point of contact on each fingertip. There are three more or less standard gaits that are characteristic of each of the doshas. They do not in and of themselves denote an imbalance. Rather, they communicate information regarding the prominence of a doshic influence.

Vata: The natural gait of vata touches the fingertips as if quickly tapping the fingers with a string. It has a swifter and more narrow or thin feeling than the gait of pitta or kapha.

Pitta: The natural gait of pitta touches the fingertips as if attempting to push them upwards with a good deal of force and definition and then drops off sharply. Typically, the gait of pitta strikes the middle of the fingertips and is of moderate breadth.

Kapha: The natural gait of kapha touches the fingertips as if water were gently swelling up from underneath or rolling across. Typically, the gait of kapha can be felt under the side of the fingertips closest to the heart. The natural gait of kapha can sometimes feel as if it begins very deep beneath the surface of the skin. It feels broad and full bodied.

In a relatively balanced rogi, the gait of the pulse will match the rogi's natural constitution throughout all the layers of the pulse.

IMBALANCES IN THE GAIT

There are many gaits of the pulse that signify specific imbalances. Generally, the pulse reader will experience some qualities of the natural dosha gait that has been "warped" to some extent or another. For instance, a pulse gait that feels like narrow pinpricks on the fingertip communicates an imbalance in the vata dosha. A pulse gait that feels like a forceful strike on the middle of the fingertip and then spreads slightly towards the sides of the point of contact communicates a pitta imbalance. A pulse gait that feels like viscous water sluggishly moving across the fingertip communicates a kapha imbalance.

The pulse reader will experience a great variety of pulse gaits throughout his or her practice. Some of them are described below.

It is imperative that the pulse reader avoids assigning a specific gait to a specific disease. The gaits found in the pulse must be taken in the context of all of the other information the pulse communicates so that the overall expression of the pulse can be discerned in its fullness.

Unlike the pulse rate, the gait is not extremely sensitive to moment-to-moment activities, times of day and emotional states. It usually takes a good deal of time and repetition of specific behaviors and reactive patterns to create a change in the gait of the pulse. This means that the pulse reader can use the gait as an indicator for more chronic disease patterns.

The pulse reader experiences imbalance in the system through the gait by reading how the gait morphs from its natural movement into a new movement.

EXAMPLES OF IMBALANCED GAITS

VATA	PITTA	KAPHA
A PINPRICK QUICKLY POKING THE FINGERTIP	STRIKES THE FINGERTIP WITH EXCESSIVE FORCE	VISCOUS WATER SLOWLY MOVING ACROSS THE FINGERTIP
A FLASH OF LIGHTING RUNNING ACROSS THE FINGERTIP	STRIKES THE FINGERTIP FORCEFULLY AND THEN SPREADS TO THE SIDES SLIGHTLY	A BARELY PERCEPTIBLE DULL BEAT, DEEP UNDER THE SURFACE OF THE SKIN, AS IF UNDERWATER
A WISP OF AIR BARELY CARESSING THE FINGERTIP	STRIKES THE FINGERTIP FORCEFULLY AND THEN STRIKES AGAIN AT ITS PEAK	PUSHES ON THE FINGERTIP AND REMAINS IN PLACE MOMENTARILY
GENTYLY TAPS THE EDGE OF THE FINGERTIP A SECOND TIME BEFORE SUBSIDING	STRIKES WITH EXCESSIVE FORCE AND THEN BALLOONS FORWARD BEFORE SUBSIDING	SPREADS OUT TO THE PERIMETER OF THE FINGERTIP IN BREADTH, AFTER MAKING INITIAL CONTACT

Dual or tridoshic imbalances can be represented in the gait. These will combine the qualities of the different gaits explained above. For example, a very broad pulse that strikes the side of the fingertip closest to the heart forcefully and then spreads towards the middle of the fingertip from the point of contact communicates a pitta-kapha imbalance.

34

The pulse reader may come across a specific kind of gait in which it will seem as though the pulse is moving backwards towards the heart. The pulse reader should investigate and pay special attention to the heart and circulatory system in this case. The pulse reader should also question the rogi as to previous or current heart conditions.

> **COMMON MISTAKE**
>
> The pulse reader can create a bias in the assessment of the gait if the pulse reading fingertips are not on the same plane. One or two fingers pushing on the pulse harder than the other(s) can create the experience of an altered gait. Unless the pulse reader is performing a specific technique in which she or he intentionally breaks the plane of the fingertips, the pulse reader should check in to make sure that proper form is being upheld.

THE FORCE AND VOLUME OF THE PULSE

The force of the pulse is a measure of how much pressure the blood is under as it flows through the veins and arteries. The pressure is determined by the volume of blood moving through a channel of a specific size. With each beat of the heart, the pressurized blood is pumped through the veins and arteries, exerting force on the vessel walls. The pulse reader can assess this force through the fingertips and thus measure a rogi's blood pressure. The more pressurized the circulatory system, the harder the heart has to work to pump blood, increasing the stress and strain on the cardiac muscle. Blood pressure is an indication of a wide variety of activities in the body and the pulse reader can become knowledgeable of these implications taken in the context of the other information communicated by the pulse.

So long as pressure is sufficient, the volume of blood moving through the radial artery determines how full or robust the pulse feels. In general, a pulse influenced primarily by vata qualities expresses less volume. A pulse influenced primarily by pitta qualities expresses a moderate volume. A pulse influenced primarily by kapha qualities expresses more volume. This is distinct from force. A pulse influenced primarily by pitta qualities exerts the highest amount of force. A pulse mostly influenced by kapha qualities exerts a moderate amount of force and a pulse influenced by vata qualities exerts the least amount of force. Commonly, the more forceful a pulse feels the more pitta's prominence is indicated. However, heavy blockages in circulatory channels or narrowing of arteries and veins can also increase the overall pressure in the system.

The pulse reader may take special note of differences between the force of the pulse on the right versus the left wrists.

If the situation allows, the pulse reader may read both radial arteries at the same time to get a clear assessment of the difference between the sides of the body. Otherwise, if the difference between sides is great enough, it will be apparent even if the left and right sides are read one after the other.

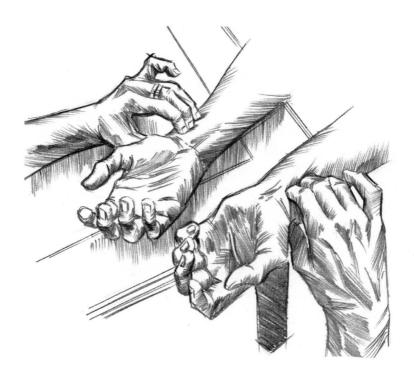

Image 14 - Reading Both Sides Simultaneously

A measure of balance in the body is indicated by a balance between the force of the pulses on both the left and right sides. It is fairly common that the pulse reader will experience an imbalance between the pulses on opposite sides of the body.

Ayurveda describes the solar and lunar channels. The primary solar channel exists in the right side of the body as the pingala. The primary lunar channel exists in the left side of the body as the ida. When the pulses are imbalanced from side to side in can indicate an imbalance in the flow of these channels and their associated functions. Here, the pulse reader should not only take into account whether the pulse is weak, but also the other qualities presenting themselves in the pulse to help determine which doshas are prominent in the imbalance.

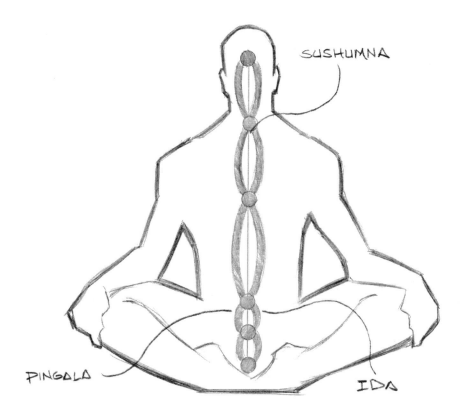

Image 15 - Pingala, Ida, and Sushumna

PINGALA

The pingala primarily governs the sympathetic nervous system. This system governs one's ability to quickly move into action from a restful state and is characterized ayurvedically as masculine. This does not mean that the sympathetic nervous system resides only on the right side of the body. Just as the heart resides on the left side of the body yet influences the entire system, the pingala resides on the right side of the body and influences the entire system. The pulse communicates information regarding the function of the pingala from the right radial artery. A weak pulse on the right side of the body can indicate a fatigued, overworked, or underperforming sympathetic nervous system.

IDA

The ida primarily governs the parasympathetic nervous system. This system governs one's ability to rest, digest and rejuvenate. It is characterized ayurvedically as feminine in quality. The pulse communicates information regarding the function of the ida from the left radial artery. A weak pulse on the left side of the body can indicate a low functioning parasympathetic nervous system which would in turn indicate issues with healing, recovery, the willingness to self-nurture or receive nurturing from others.

If either the ida or pingala is out of balance, then the other one will also not function well. The same goes for the parasympathetic and sympathetic nervous systems. For instance, a digestive imbalance can be caused by either or both nervous systems going out of balance. It is likely the case that both systems will need re-balancing simultaneously and in context with one another.

The pulse reader's intention is to look beyond the immediate symptoms and discern from where the issue is stemming, the root cause.

In this manner, regardless of whether both systems need re-balancing, the pulse reader can identify in which system the imbalance began and continues to be perpetuated from. The inability to eliminate the root cause of an imbalance may allow for temporary relief of symptoms, but not complete restoration of harmony in the rogi's body.

The pulse reader must also pay attention to the obvious when it comes to pulse imbalances from side-to-side. Namely, the imbalance of the circulatory system. If the pulse is extremely weak from one side to the other, then the pulse reader should investigate the cardiac and circulatory systems further. Vital blockages in the circulatory system may be present.

COMMON MISTAKE

Much like rate and rhythm, it is easy for the pulse reader to forget that the time of day, rogi's emotional state, and the rogi's activities immediately preceding the pulse reading greatly affect the force of the pulse. The force of the pulse is highly changeable on a moment-to-moment basis.

SURFACE-TEMPERATURE AND TEXTURE OF THE SKIN AND RADIAL ARTERY

The combination of the surface temperature of the skin and texture of the skin serve two more sources of information for the pulse reader. While not directly related to the pulse itself, the qualities presented by the skin will be ascertained in the process of reading the pulse. There are a few qualities that are particularly revealing upon touching the skin. The first is body temperature. The surface of the skin could feel hot, warm, cool or cold. The second is the texture of the skin. It could be smooth, clammy, rough, dry, brittle or a combination of different textures. Each of these qualities contribute to the overall discernment that the pulse reader is working towards. Hot, dry skin would indicate pitta and vata imbalances while cold and clammy skin would indicate a kapha or potentially pitta and kapha imbalances.

The temperature of the skin reveals a good deal of information about the nature of the circulatory system. Cool or warm skin is not an indication of imbalance, but excessively hot or excessively cold skin may be. If either of these extremes are felt on the surface temperature of the skin the pulse reader should pay extra notice to the functions of the circulatory system, including the heart and diaphragm. For example, if the skin is very hot, the heart rate is high and the breath rate is quickened, then there is a heavy indication that pitta is highly active which could then force vata to behave irregularly while simultaneously destroying the healthy qualities of kapha. The rogi may display symptoms like hyperacidity, rashes, agitated behavior and the like.

If the skin is very cold, the heart rate is low and the breath rate is very slow, then there is a heavy indication that kapha is highly active which could then block the natural flow of vata and snuff out the healthy qualities of pitta. The rogi may display symptoms such as excess mucous, low appetite, depressive behavior and the like.

The other texture to take note of is that of the artery itself. The pulse reader can ascertain how elastic, resilient, tough or feeble the radial artery feels by applying pressure to it. The pulse reader must take into account how much muscle, fat and skin cover the artery itself as this will greatly influence the feeling that the pulse reader experiences when applying pressure. For instance, an obese rogi's radial artery will be covered by more adipose tissue giving the pulse a deeper feeling. The pulse reader must take this into account and not mistake this with the type of depth that is felt when reading the pulse of a rogi with a kapha prominent constitution. Sensitizing one's self to feeling the quality of the vessel wall itself is a technique that requires practice over time and exposure to a wide range of individuals' pulses.

COMMON MISTAKE

The pulse reader must learn his or her own day-to-day surface skin temperature. If the pulse reader usually feels hot, a rogi's skin who runs just as hot may only feel warm.

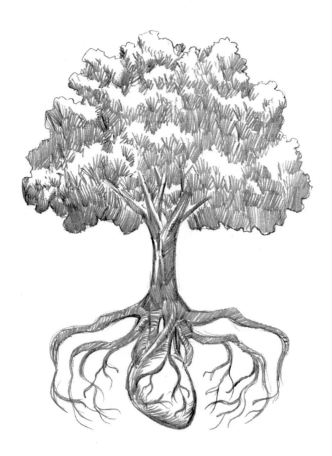

Image 16 - The Pulse of Nature

CHAPTER FOUR

CONTACT POINTS ON THE FINGERTIPS, LAYERS, AND PREPARING TO DELVE DEEPER

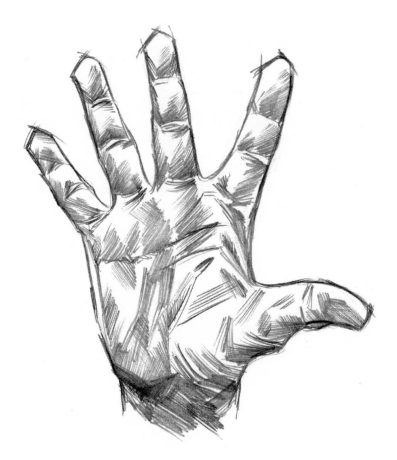

Image 17 - Locations of Contact

The pulse is felt on up to five points on each the index, middle and ring fingers. Depending on which layer of the pulse the pulse reader is observing, she or he will observe either *three* or *five* of these points.

THREE LOCATIONS OF CONTACT

On layers in which the pulse reader feels for *three* contact points on each of the fingertips, the *kapha* location is the first third of the fingertip closest to the rogi's heart, the *pitta* location is the middle third of the fingertip, and the *vata* location is the third of the fingertip furthest from the rogi's heart.

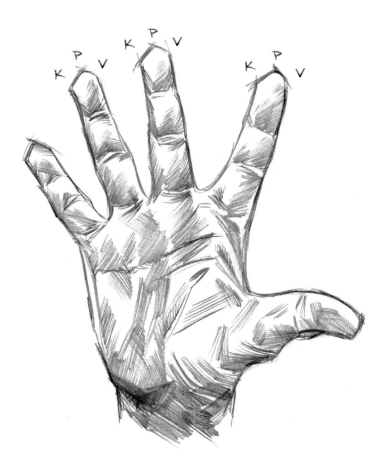

Image 18 - Three Locations of Contact

Victor Briere A.D.

AN IMPORTANT NOTE ON ANNOTATIONS

In the remaining chapters, where relevant, the overall doshic qualities expressed by each crest will be indicated by the first letter of the appropriate dosha. *These annotations represent the qualities being expressed and __not__ the location of the crests.* The below image serves as an example. The "P" under the crest indicates that pitta *qualities* are being expressed through the pulse. The point of contact is on the vata *location* of the fingertip.

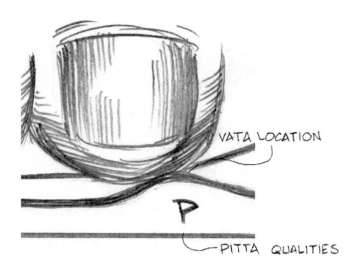

Image 19 - Crest Location and Crest Qualities

There are two factors that the pulse reader must always consider. First is the location(s) on each fingertip where the crest of the pulse is experienced. Second is the qualities expressed by each crest.

This does __not__ necessarily mean that the pulse reader will experience kapha *qualities* at the kapha *location*, the third of the fingertip closest to the heart. The points of contact are identified by dosha because these are the natural locations for each dosha to express themselves

44

on each fingertip. Vata qualities expressing themselves at the vata location of the fingertip is more of an indication of balance than vata qualities expressing themselves at the kapha location of the same fingertip.

The exception to this is in the prakruti layer. A pitta prominent individual may have pulses that express pitta qualities on every location. In such cases, the pulse reader should measure the other layers by the qualities found in the prakruti and not the "natural" locations of each crest. For example, a pitta prominent individual expressing all pitta qualities on the prakruti layer would still be considered to have an imbalance if vata is expressing its qualities on the third of the fingertip furthest from the heart on the index finger in the vikruti layer.

The student of the pulse may find it most convenient and simple to assess the entire pulse in the context of the prakruti and use the doshic labels of the fingertip locations mainly as a naming device. However, this aspect of pulse reading should not be forgotten completely, as qualities that neither match the prakruti, nor are found in their natural location, will certainly inform the pulse reader of bodily dysfunction.

FIVE LOCATIONS OF CONTACT

The *only* layer in which the pulse reader takes five points of contact into account is the third layer of the pulse. This is the layer in which subdoshic activity is read. There are five subdoshas of each dosha. Each of the five points corresponds to a different subdosha. The ring fingertip reads the kapha subdoshas, the middle fingertip reads the pitta subdoshas and the index fingertip reads the vata subdoshas.

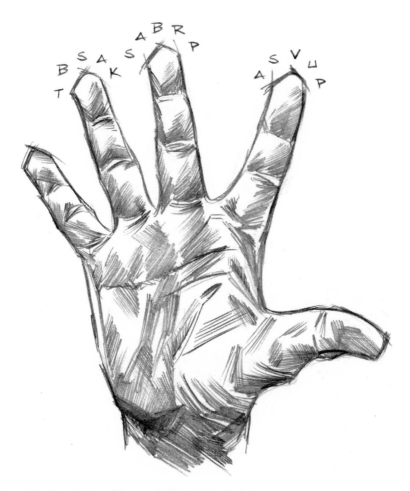

Image 20 - Five Points of Contact for the Subdosha Layer

OVERALL

Again, on every layer of the pulse, regardless of where the pulse crests on each fingertip, the quality of the pulse must be taken into account.

The pulse reader will experience that the pulse crests at different locations on each of the fingertips on different layers. The crest's change in location on each of the fingertips from layer to layer is created by the varying amounts of pressure that the pulse reader exerts on the radial artery, in relationship to the nature of the rogi's pulse. This is the way in which the pulse reader "prompts" or "asks" the pulse to provide different information regarding the body. In this sense, the pulse reader enters into a truly unique kind of *conversation* with the body. The pulse reader asks "questions" by moving between layers and the pulse "responds" by changing the location and qualitative patterns it expresses from layer to layer.

Each fingertip can, and will likely, experience crests in different locations on the same layer. Some crests will contact the same location on a fingertip for multiple layers before suddenly changing to a different location. Some crests will contact the same location on the same fingertip throughout all of the layers of the pulse. Some crests will change location on every layer. It will be completely different from rogi to rogi. When combined with the fact that each expression on each layer on each location of each fingertip can express its own qualities, it becomes apparent that there are thousands of permutations and combinations that can be potentially expressed.

COMMON MISTAKE

Many pulse readers tilt their hand laterally while delving into or ascending from different layers. When this happens, the fingertips change their orientation to the pulse from centered to skewed. This creates a bias in which the pulse reader feels the crest of the pulse on a point of the fingertip that he or she wouldn't have otherwise. It is similar to misunderstanding what someone means in a conversation due to a personal bias carried by the listener.

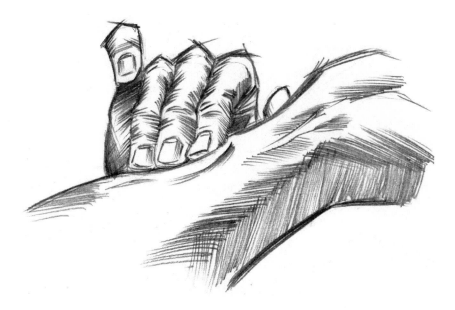

Image 21 - Skewed, Incorrect, Finger Placement

MULTIPLE CRESTS ON ONE FINGERTIP

It is common, especially in the third layer and deeper, that the pulse reader will feel two crests making contact on a single fingertip in different locations. It is often the case that they will be of similar quality and on polar sides of the fingertip. In these cases, both locations and their respective corollaries are being expressed.

The pulse reader may also experience a definite prominence of one crest at one location and a more subtle crest in a different location on the same fingertip. This can be very easy to miss. Sometimes, a crest will be so prominent that it drowns out the feeling of other crests that are more moderate but still conveying information.

A double crest on one fingertip is distinct from the gait of the pulse. The gait of the pulse expresses itself within each individual crest. It is common to find the same gait repeated over and over in each individual crest.

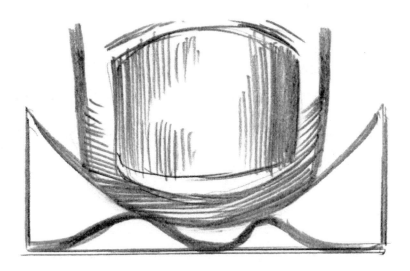

Image 22 - Two Crests Making Contact on One Fingertip

LAYERS OF THE PULSE

In this style of pulse reading seven layers are used to prompt the pulse to provide information. Accessing each layer is a matter of applying a refined amount of pressure to the radial artery, evenly distributed across the plane of the pulse reading fingers. Unless reading the organ pulses, the pulse reading fingers move through the layers as a single unit.

This is the basic chart that will be used to depict reading the pulse on different layers in later chapters. The fingers and pulse will be shown on each layer along with examples of different crest patterns. The ring finger will be depicted as the left-most finger.

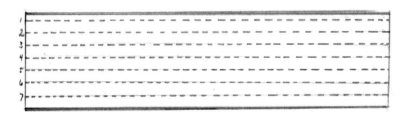

Image 23 - Basic Pulse Layer Annotation

49

DELVING DEEPER - LISTENING

The body is a highly intelligent organism. It possesses an intelligence that is not immediately perceptible to our everyday sensory experiences. Within this intelligence is an extremely sophisticated ability to communicate within itself and the environment around it. The body can be likened to one who speaks multiple languages with perfect accentuation in many different dialects. The pulse reader doesn't just learn one of the body's languages. Rather, she or he learns how to interpret one of the body's continuous expressions. The body's pulse of life is present from the 24th day of pregnancy up until the moment of death.

The pulse reader's primary motivation is to *listen* while the body *expresses*. It is a communication in its truest form. When someone is speaking, the listener doesn't take the words for their meaning at face value. The words are put into the *context* of the entire expression of the speaker. Only a poor or distracted listener takes the meaning of spoken words as a literal and complete expression of what is being *communicated.*

Listening is not being used as a metaphor for a deeper meaning of touch. While the pulse reader is using the sense of touch to receive the pulse's expression, the pulse reader is using the capacity of listening to understand the body's communication.

This is a vital recognition for the pulse reader. Each sense organ, when united with the mind through focused awareness, creates a different sensory experience than is not present otherwise. Hearing becomes *listening*. Touching becomes *feeling*. Looking becomes *seeing*. Tasting becomes *savoring*. Smelling becomes *recognition*. This description of the senses is not a poetic device. It is an ayurvedic description of the functional and physiological changes that occur when the mind unites with a particular sense organ. While extraordinarily fast, the mind can technically only unite with one sense organ at a time. Knowing this, the pulse reader maintains her or his focus on uniting the mind first with touch to truly *feel* the pulse and then immediately after unites the mind with hearing to truly *listen* to the expression of the pulse and understand the meaning of its expression.

Listening is one's capacity to deeply understand the essence of an expression.

It is through listening that the pulse reader interprets his or her own experience of the pulse. Listening is a function of the akash element, expansive and omnipresent. While listening, the pulse reader consciously enhances the qualities of akash in the mind. This allows the pulse reader to perceive the full expression of the rogi's pulse. Amidst the fullness of that expression, the pulse reader's *intuition* perceives knowledge of both the body as a whole and its different aspects.

This is where the pulse reader needs to pay special attention to him or herself and the quality of the mind. Whenever the mind unites with a sense organ it brings along with it biases or baggage it carries. The pulse reader may receive touch information but not listen to what is being conveyed. Or, the pulse reader may receive touch information and interpret something that isn't there. The pulse reader must learn to cultivate a neutrality while reading pulses in order to avoid such biases. The primary qualities of the neutrality are to:

1) Remain in the present and not project a pre-determined outcome onto the present
2) Engage a compassionate attitude that is not concerned with judging one's self or the rogi
3) Deeply discern the truth via listening
4) Responding as opposed to reacting

CHAPTER FIVE

PRAKRUTI
THE SEVENTH LAYER
OF THE PULSE

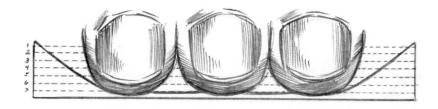

Image 24 - The Seventh Layer

The prakruti is the balanced form and function of an individual. It is the individual's natural constitution. Contained within it is the individual's ideal, unique doshic and elemental recipe. An individual's prakruti is found on the deepest layer of the pulse, the seventh layer, and is assessed via three points of contact on each of the fingertips.

A pulse reader's ability to accurately ascertain an individual's prakruti creates a context for all other information the pulse reader discerns.

For example, a slow heart rate with skin that is cool to the touch in the context of a kapha prominent prakruti is a sign of balance. The same information in the context of a pitta prominent prakruti can indicate a sign of imbalance.

While reading this layer of the pulse *often* communicates a rogi's prakruti, it does not *always* communicate the rogi's prakruti. It is possible for imbalances in the pulse to be present on this layer as well as every other layer. This typically occurs when the rogi is severely imbalanced, suffering from life-threatening diseases such as cancer or highly debilitating diseases such as muscular dystrophy.

To read the seventh layer of the pulse, begin at the first layer. From the first layer, apply pressure on the radial artery until the pulse is completely stopped. It is not always possible to stop the pulse completely. In these cases, the pulse reader may apply pressure until the pulse is only felt on the kapha point of contact on the ring finger. From this position, release the pressure just enough to allow the pulse to flow underneath all three fingertips. *This is the seventh layer of the pulse.*

Below is an example of what the pulse reader may experience. Reading the diagram from left to right, the ring fingertip is contacted by the pulse on the kapha and vata locations, the middle finger on the pitta location and the index finger on the kapha and vata locations.

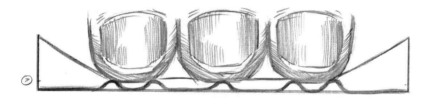

Image 25 - Example of a Prakruti Pulse

If the qualities were to match the locations, then this would be an example of a vata/kapha prominent prakruti. If the qualities were to differ from crest to crest, or if the crests were expressing primarily pitta qualities, then the pulse reader would need to discern what he or she believes to be the most prominent force acting in the body. There are as many prakrutis as there are people. While it is convenient to label them in terms of doshic categories, the reality of the prakruti is unique to each individual.

NATURAL LOCATIONS OF THE DOSHAS

Kapha's natural location is under the ring finger on the heart side, pitta's is in the middle of the middle finger, and vata is on the thumb's side of the index finger. Finding a crest in its natural location on the prakruti layer represents that the dosha is functioning exceedingly smoothly.

This does <u>not</u> mean that there is an imbalance in the prakruti layer of the pulse simply because the doshas are not represented in their natural locations. It is extremely common for the representation of the doshas in the pulse to be found outside of their natural locations. This is what creates a wide variety of prakrutis.

Each dosha and its corresponding qualities can potentially be felt by any fingertip, in any location.

However, when a dosha is represented in its natural location it often acts as an anchor in the prakruti, or an especially organizing force for the constitution. On the seventh layer, when a dosha is represented in its natural location, it communicates a stability and resilience associated with that dosha's functioning within the body.

EXAMPLE OF A SEVENTH LAYER PULSE

As depicted below, the constitution is dominantly pitta, but pitta is also in its natural location, in the middle of the middle finger. However, kapha and vata are also in their natural locations even though there is a pitta crest on both the ring and index fingers as well. This does not mean that pitta is imbalanced because it is also felt outside its natural location. Imbalance is read by comparing the other layers of the pulse, especially the first layer, to the prakruti. Kapha and vata are functioning at a high level of stability in the system but pitta is leading the function of the system due to its prominence throughout the pulse. This is an example of an extremely stable prakruti.

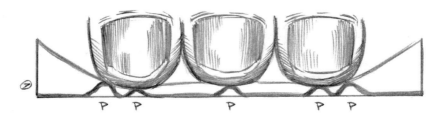

Image 26 - Example of a Seventh Layer Pulse

COMMON MISTAKE

Some pulse readers make the understandable error of confusing a seriously ill rogi's seventh layer pulse as the proper representation of the prakruti. If a rogi is presenting severe, potentially life-threatening symptoms then the pulse becomes so compromised that even the seventh layer becomes impaired. In such cases, prakruti cannot be read in the pulse until the rogi has recovered to some degree.

55

CHAPTER SIX

VIKRUTI
THE FIRST LAYER OF THE PULSE

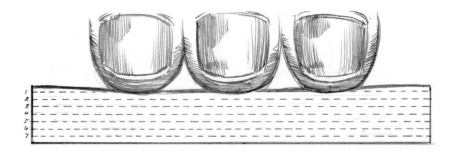

Image 27 - The First Layer

Vikruti is an individual's doshic patterning and behavior up to and *including the present moment*. It is used to assess how far the functioning of the body has strayed from prakruti, and thus is used to measure imbalance in the body. The vikruti pulse is felt on the first layer by placing the fingertips on the radial artery *very* lightly, hardly depressing the skin at all. The only exception to this is if the rogi is overweight and the pulse cannot be felt with such a light touch. In this case the pulse reader may apply more pressure, without breaking the plane of the fingertips, up to the point where the pulse on any of the fingertips first presents itself.

When the vikruti pulse matches the prakruti pulse in both location and quality, the individual is balanced.

This is a rare condition in the modern world but true, nevertheless. A matching vikruti and prakruti indicates that the ideal form and function of the body is pervading through all of its layers, dhatus, doshas and organs. It is not a rare occurrence just because of the modern, imbalanced lifestyle. Vikruti can change from moment to moment. The pulse reader must remember, that the doshas are continuously changing their status in relationship with each other based on time, season, climate, phase of life, food intake, water intake, perceptual experience, sexual activity, emotional state, etc.

COMMON MISTAKE

The pulse reader will very lightly place her or his fingertips on the vikruti pulse but will not experience a pulse on the ring fingertip at all. To compensate for this, the pulse reader will apply more pressure to the radial artery. This actually sends the pulse reader into a deeper layer of the pulse and is no longer reading of the vikruti. The lack of a particular pulse on the first layer, commonly, but not exclusively, the ring fingertip pulse, is a sign of imbalance. Typically, it indicates a generalized depletion in the body affecting the overall force and volume of the pulse.

EXAMPLE OF A FIRST LAYER PULSE

To know how the pulse is expressing vikruti, the pulse reader must know what the prakruti is. In the below example the location of the pitta crest on the ring fingertip matches, but there is no expression of the kapha crest on the ring finger as in the prakruti. The middle finger in the vikruti layer has no expression of pitta, instead, it is expressing kapha and vata crests. Finally, the pitta crest matches that of the prakruti but there is an absence of the vata crest. By the location of the crests alone, the pulse reader can ascertain that both the vata and kapha doshas, and to some extent the pitta dosha, are functioning irregularly.

VIKRUTI – LAYER ONE

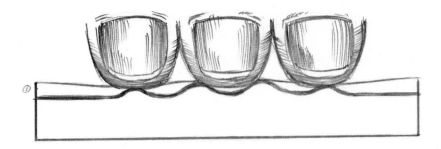

Image 28 - Example of a First Layer Pulse

PRAKRUTI – LAYER SEVEN

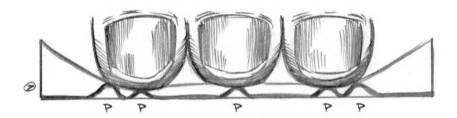

Image 29 - Example of a Prakruti Pulse for Determining Vikruti

In the pulse reader's self-talk, he or she will also discern the qualities that each crest is expressing. This will fill out the nature of the imbalances. For example, if the crests under the ring, middle and index fingertips are expressing vata qualities, while in the prakruti they express pitta or kapha qualities, the pulse reader can begin to understand that the general nature of the imbalance will be mostly associated, at its root, with the improper functioning of vata. Which in turn, may be warping the functioning of kapha and pitta. In this case, the pulse reader can pay extra attention to irregular vata crests throughout all the layers of the pulse.

If instead the crest under the ring, middle and index fingertips are expressing kapha qualities while the crests on the prakruti layer are expressing pitta and/or vata qualities, then the pulse reader can begin to understand that the general nature of the imbalance will be mostly associated, at its root, with the improper function of kapha and then influencing pitta and vata thereafter.

It is common that qualities representing two or three of the doshas are expressed by different crests on different fingers. The pulse may express vata qualities through the ring fingertip crest, pitta qualities through the middle fingertip crests and kapha qualities through the index fingertip crest, all of which are different than that which is expressed on the prakruti level. It is up to the pulse reader to translate the significance of all of these expressions in the context of the prakruti and all the other layers of the pulse. The pulse reader will encounter a seemingly endless number of permutations and combinations of crest locations and qualities.

While this may seem daunting at first, revelations of salient features and patterns begin to unfold effortlessly within the pulse reader as her or his perception and intuition becomes more refined.

The information attained from reading the prakruti pulse and vikruti pulse alone is enough to go great lengths in the understanding of imbalance in an individual's body. The vikruti yields immediately relevant, generalized, systemic knowledge that can inform the pulse reader which dosha and functions require aid in a holistic sense.

CHAPTER SEVEN

GETTING MORE SPECIFIC – THE SUBDOSHAS THE THIRD LAYER OF THE PULSE

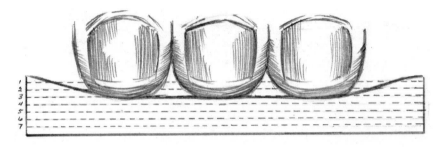

Image 30 - The Third Layer

Vata, pitta and kapha form the basic intelligences from which the subdoshas emerge. The subdoshas are divisions of vata, pitta and kapha that perform different functions in the body. Each is specialized and has a particular region or regions of function. Each subdosha also has a site of origin from which it performs its primary function.

The pulse reader experiences the subdoshas in the pulse by observing all five locations on each of the fingertips. The subdoshas of kapha are read on the ring fingertip, those of pitta on the middle fingertip and those of vata on the index fingertip. The presence of a crest does not necessarily represent imbalance in the activity of a subdosha. Rather, it expresses which of the subdoshas are most active in the present moment. For this reason, the crests do <u>not</u> need to match the prakruti to represent balance in the body.

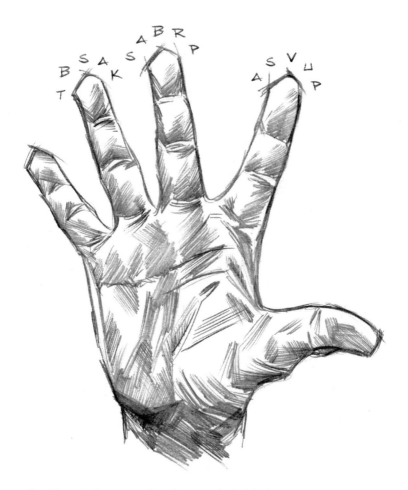

Image 31 - Fingertip Locations Correlating to the Subdoshas

The subdoshas offer a wonderful opportunity for the pulse reader to practice on him or herself. Just before a bowel movement, the pulse reader may find that apana is very active. Just after, the pulse reader may find one of the other vata subdoshas to be most active. Just after practicing pranayama, prana vata may likely be active. Just after eating, kledaka kapha may be active. Just after working on a computer for some time, alochaka pitta may be active. The pulse reader can learn the rhythms of her or his body very intimately by engaging the third layer of the pulse. Practicing on one's self makes it easier to identify common subdoshic patterns in others.

61

THE SUBDOSHAS, THEIR SITES OF ORIGIN AND PRIMARY FUNCTION

VATA	PRANA	UDANA	VYANA	SAMANA	APANA
ORIGIN	HEART	LUNGS	HEART	INTESTINES	COLON
MOVEMENT	INWARD	OUT AND UP	CENTRIFUGAL	LINEAR	OUT AND DOWN
PITTA	PACHAKA	RANJAKA	BHRAJAKA	ALOCHAKA	SADHAKA
ORIGIN	STOMACH	LIVER	SKIN	EYES	HEART AND BRAIN
FUNCTION	TO COOK	TO COLOR	TO REGULATE	TO SEE	TO DISCERN
KAPHA	KLEDAKA	AVALAMBAKA	SHLESHAKA	BODHAKA	TARPAKA
ORIGIN	STOMACH	LUNGS AND HEART	JOINTS	MOUTH	BRAIN
FUNCTION	TO MOISTEN	TO ENVELOP	TO BIND	TO KNOW	TO NOURISH

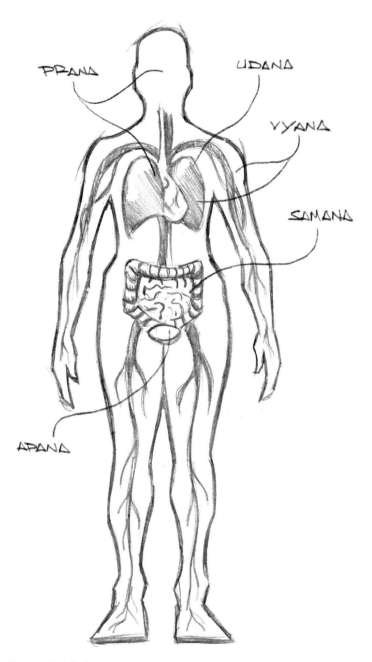

Image 32 - Vata Subdoshas

VATA SUBDOSHAS

Vata is the only dosha that moves. The other two and their subdoshas are inert and completely rely on the force of vata to move throughout the body. Vata's subdoshas create pressure and flow in the body.

In particular, the vata subdoshas are highly sensitive to each other's functions because vata flows continuously through every part of the body. If apana is blocked, and elimination isn't balanced, there is a high likelihood that all of the subdoshas of vata will become imbalanced to some degree. The same goes for the other subdoshas in relation to each other to a lesser degree.

Vata is a continuous flow. If a channel is blocked, damaged or severed then vata will change its course. In time, this can change the form and function of the dhatus, organs and the doshas within them. This is a cause for many chronic imbalances.

Prana vata governs the inward motions. Its primary functions are the intake of food, water, sense perceptions, and breath.

Udana vata governs the upward and outward motions. Its primary functions are exhalation and expressions such as speech. Udana vata has a direct relationship with physical strength and outward exertion.

Vyana vata governs the centrifugal motion. Its primary function is to circulate fluids, including blood, throughout the body.

Samana vata governs the "linear" motions of peristalsis through the intestines. Its primary function is to separate nourishment from waste and harmonize all of the subdoshas doshas involved in digestion.

Apana vata governs the downward and outward motions. Its primary functions are the evacuation of both urine and feces as well as the secretion of different fluids from their respective organs throughout the body.

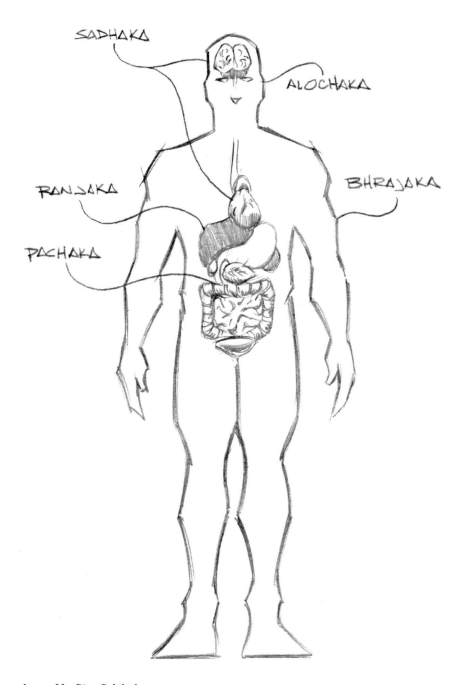

Image 33 - Pitta Subdoshas

PITTA SUBDOSHAS

Pitta's subdoshas digest and transform both substances and perceptions into bodily tissues and fluids. Pitta is the primary dosha involved in the strength and function of agni. Its subdoshas are different functions of agni within the whole.

Pachaka pitta governs digestive fluids within their respective organs. Its seat is in the stomach and duodenum.

Ranjaka pitta governs the coloring of blood, urine and feces. Its seat is in the liver.

Bhrajaka pitta governs temperature regulation of the overall body and the transfer of substances through the skin. Its seat is in the skin.

Alochaka pitta governs the sense of sight and the interpretation of images within the eyes. Its seat is in the eyes.

Sadhaka pitta governs the digestion of sense perceptions and information moving through the nervous system. As such it plays an important role in intellect and discernment. Its seat is in the heart and secondarily in the brain.

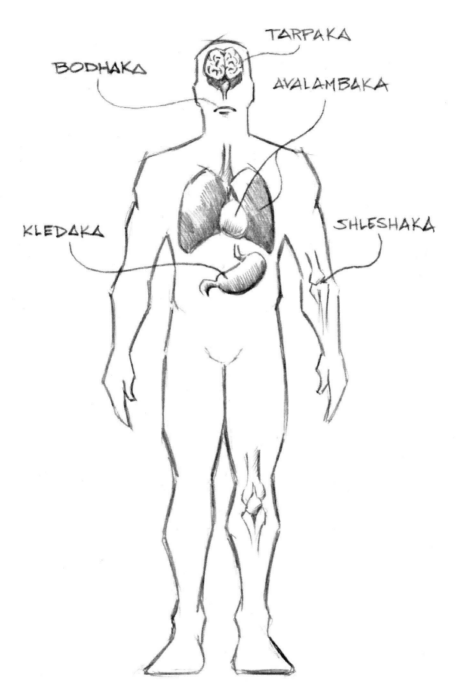

Image 34 - Kapha Subdoshas

KAPHA SUBDOSHAS

Kapha's subdoshas protect the dhatus and form the containers from which both pitta and vata fulfill their functions. The kapha subdoshas each have a protective aspect to them. They not only form the containers for the other doshas but provide protection against the excess influences of that which they contain.

Kledaka kapha governs the linings in the stomach. It combines with food in the stomach to protect the nourishment within food from being overexposed to hydrochloric acid. It also protects the stomach tissue from overexposure to hydrochloric acid. Its seat is in the stomach.

Avalambaka kapha governs the linings in and around the lungs as well as the pericardium. It is liquid in nature and highly protective, acting as a sort of shock absorber for the heart and lungs which are in constant motion. Its presence in the lungs is necessary to keep them from drying out due to the constant exposure to the movements of vata via respiration. Its primary seat is in the lungs and heart.

Shleshaka kapha governs the lubrication fluids found in the joints. These fluids ensure that the bones do not damage themselves via friction. Its seat is in the joints.

Bodhaka kapha governs saliva. It contains digestive enzymes created by pitta to initialize the digestive process in the mouth. It also protects the tissues of the mouth from overexposure to vata. It is necessary for the sense of taste as taste buds only operate when they are moist. Its seat is in the mouth.

Tarpaka kapha governs cerebrospinal fluid, grey brain matter and white brain matter. It is full of nourishment to contain, protect and vitalize the majja dhatu. Its seat is in the brain.

TIMING AND THE THIRD LAYER

Due to the constantly changing nature of subdoshic activity, it is beneficial if the pulse reader can take a rogi's pulse on multiple occasions, at different times, over the course of days, months and years. In this way the pulse reader can learn that particular rogi's subdoshic tendencies. If for example, avalambaka kapha, bhrajaka pitta and apana vata is active in every pulse reading performed, there likely exists some kind of imbalance in the skin. In this case avalambaka kapha could signal the pulse reader that the rogi is under a good deal of emotional stress, bhrajaka pitta is a direct correlate to the skin and apana vata indicates challenges with elimination. All of these combined point to a high likelihood of rashes, eruptions, skin discoloration etc.

The pulse reader should also take note of what time of day and what activities the rogi performed just before the pulse reading. In a balanced body, subdoshas are commonly active before, during, and after activities that correspond to their function. If the pulse is read just before the rogi eats lunch to find an active pachaka pitta pulse would not be surprising. However, if during the same time, apana vata is high, and there is a very feeble pachaka pitta pulse expressing vata qualities via its crest, then it is a very strong indication that the rogi's digestive fire is impaired due to constipation or a related issue

EXAMPLE OF A THIRD LAYER PULSE

The pulse is cresting on the ring fingertip on the avalambaka kapha and tarpaka kapha locations, the middle finger on the ranjaka pitta location and the index finger on the samana vata location. This means that bodhaka kapha, kledaka kapha, alochaka pitta and udana vata are all active in the body at the present moment.

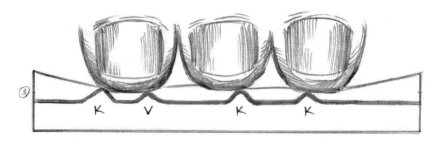

Image 35 - Example of a Third Layer Pulse

This could be a subdoshic pattern found just after a rogi has eaten ice cream to compensate for emotional stress, especially if the qualities expressed through the crests are kapha and/or vata in nature. Two of the kapha subdoshas are active. Avalambaka kapha is extremely sensitive to an individual's emotional states and stress levels. The activity of tarpaka kapha indicates fluids moving towards the brain and through the spine as a result of a high dosage of sugar in response to emotional stress. Ranjaka pitta is often active just after an individual has eaten and the liver is processing blood, producing and secreting digestive enzymes. Samana vata is also often active just after an individual eats, increasing peristalsis in the intestines. The kapha qualities found in the crests are present due to the influence of the cold quality and sweet taste of ice cream. The vata qualities were present prior to the rogi eating due to the high stress levels.

If the rogi were to have a vata prominent prakruti, and a kapha prominent vikruti, then the third layer of the pulse is the detailed storyteller explaining why this is the case.

COMMON MISTAKE

Many pulse readers isolate the information received regarding the subdoshas to their corresponding systems, dhatus and organs. For example, an imbalance in apana to the large intestine. Information ascertained from the subdosha expressions should never be taken alone. It needs to be synthesized with the functioning of the other subdoshas to form a more holistic picture of activity within the body

---

CHAPTER EIGHT

THE DHATUS
THE FIFTH LAYER OF THE PULSE

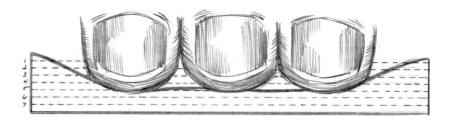

Image 36 - The Fifth Layer

The seven dhatus are the different tissues that make up the physical form. While each dhatu is spread throughout the body, they each have primary sites of creation and evacuation. Each dhatu, except majja and shukra/arthava, has what is called an 'upadhatu' which is a sub-tissue of the main tissue. All of the dhatus except shukra/arthava have 'malas' which are bi-products of the creation of that tissue. Many call these bi-products waste, but in fact they have functions of their own. For example, finger and toenails are one of the malas of asthi. It would be folly to say they are simply waste and provide no function.

Dosha aggravation alone cannot produce a disease. It merely produces a temporary, aggravated state. The aggravation must localize in a weakened dhatu to take root and progress as a disease.

All dhatus are intimately connected with each other, the organs, and doshas, and should not be assessed in isolation. They function together and they nourish each other. Strictly speaking, there is never just an imbalance in one dhatu alone without any influence on any other part of the body. It is tempting to categorize and organize functions and form for ease of understanding and communication, but, above all, the pulse reader is seeking to perceive the truth that lies beyond this convenience.

The pulse reader observes the dhatus on the fifth layer of the pulse on three locations. The same locations as in the prakruti and vikruti. The kapha location on the ring finger represents the rasa dhatu, the pitta location the shukra dhatu, and the vata location the rakta dhatu. The kapha location on the middle finger represents the mamsa dhatu, the pitta location the shukra dhatu again, and the vata location the meda dhatu. The kapha location on the index finger represents the asthi dhatu, the pitta location the shukra dhatu once more, and the vata location the majja dhatu. The below image depicts this.

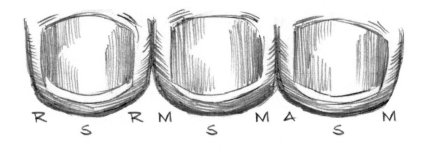

Image 37 - Dhatus on the Fingertips

The fifth layer need not mirror the prakruti in location. An overall difference in the qualities expressed in this layer in comparison to the prakruti layer should be noted. Part of what determines the formation of a dhatu is the nature of the prakruti. The location of the crests found in the fifth layer of the pulse show activity in the dhatu. The qualities expressed via the crests communicate which doshas are most influentially acting on the dhatu in the present moment. The pulse reader could find expressions of any of the three doshas on any fingertip on any location.

The pulse reader should take note when the doshic influence caries the opposite qualities of the prakruti in relation to the dhatu. This is a potential sign of imbalance.

Unlike the third layer, patterns in the dhatu pulse tend not to change as quickly. The quickest dhatus to change are rasa and rakta and in some cases shukra/arthava. It can take over a month for patterns to change in the asthi, majja and shukra/arthava pulses as these dhatus take a longer period of time for the body to generate via the digestive process.

Dhatus are constituents. For example, mamsa is not muscle, it is the substance out of which muscle is created. Meda is not fat, it is the substance out of which fat is created, and so on...

Given this, the pulse reader should not be baffled by an expression of excess kapha in the meda dhatu while sitting in front of a person with a balanced body weight and balanced muscle tone. The meda dhatu is responsible for many other types of fluids in the body such as synovial fluid. The imbalance found in the pulse may lie in those.

Each dhatu has a site of origin and a site of removal. Issues with these sites can create challenges with the dhatu agnis. Dhatu agni is the body's ability to digest and transform elemental constituents into each individual dhatu. If the primary agni is low, then dhatu agnis will be affected. If the pulse reader comes across an expression of imbalance in a dhatu pulse one of its corresponding sites and a subdosha related to that site or dhatu, then a major portion of the pathology has been illuminated.

For example, on the fifth layer, the pulse reader experiences that rakta is active with a pitta prominent crest. On the third layer, the pulse reader experiences that ranjaka pitta is active, with kapha qualities expressed in the crest. The pulse reader then checks the liver pulse to find that it is weak with kapha qualities being expressed through the crest as well. The liver is the site of origin for rakta and the primary seat of ranjaka pitta. There is a strong indication that the liver function is sluggish and unable to generate or purify blood properly. The pitta qualities in the blood are not being balanced, leading to an issue with the rakta dhatu. To take the example one step further, if the rogi were to develop gout and then later arthritis in the same location, the pulse reader can see the samprapti playing

73

out via the layers of the pulse, ultimately resulting in damage to the asthi dhatu.

If the fifth layer of the pulse is feeble overall, and there are no obvious crests in the pulse, it is an indication that agni throughout the entire body is weak.

Each of the dhatus are represented below with a few examples of how imbalances in the dhatus, upadhatus and malas may express themselves in the pulse and body for each dosha. *This, by no means is an exhaustive list of imbalances that arise from compromised dhatus.* Many of the below examples can be caused by sophisticated mixtures of doshas, subdoshas and dhatus. The examples serve as a tool for the student to practice synthesizing the qualities expressed in the fifth layer with the other layers of the pulse.

RASA DHATU

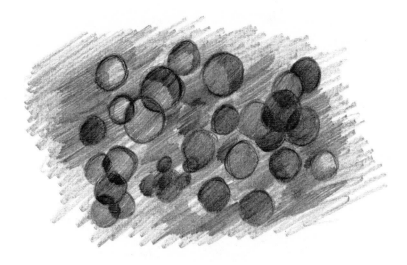

Image 38 - Rasa Dhatu

Rasa dhatu is the first dhatu created via the digestion of food and liquids. It is created in the heart and the veins/arteries stemming from the heart. It is evacuated primarily through the top layer of the skin, the kidneys and feces. Most of rasa is used to directly

74

nourish the other dhatus. As such there is no upadhatu in men, and only temporary upadhatus in women in the form of breast milk and menstrual fluid. The mala is the kapha dosha itself.

If the pulse reader experiences imbalanced kapha qualities anywhere in the pulse, but especially expressed in the rasa dhatu crest, it could mean that the rasa dhatu is producing too much of its mala creating any condition associated with excess kapha. This is one of the primary indicators of both ama and weakened agni. In such cases the rogi may also suffer from kapha related menstrual disorders such as clotting because menstrual blood is one of the upadhatus of rasa. Since the mala may be too abundant, the pulse reader should pay special attention to the organ of creation, the heart, and the organs of evacuation, the skin and kidneys.

If the pulse reader experiences imbalanced vata qualities in the rasa dhatu pulse, it could mean that the rasa dhatu is depleted. This creates depletion of all the other dhatus. The pulse reader may also inquire about the upadhatu which may indicate amenorrhea, menstrual cramps or lack of breast milk production in new mothers.

If the pulse reader experiences imbalanced pitta qualities anywhere in the pulse, but especially expressed in the rasa dhatu crest, it could mean that agni is too strong, destroying the nutrition contained within rasa dhatu. The difference between the pitta and vata imbalance is that in the former, the depletion is occurring via the destruction of rasa. In the latter the depletion is occurring because of a lack of production of rasa. Excess pitta in the rasa dhatu can also create depletion of all the other dhatus or the improper formation of the rakta dhatu. The upadhatu may express itself as odorous menstrual discharge and yellow tinged breast milk.

RAKTA DHATU

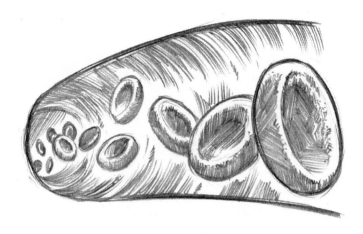

Image 39 - Rakta Dhatu

Rakta dhatu is the constituent that creates red blood cells. It is completely intermixed with rasa dhatu in the veins and arteries. It is created primarily by the liver and recycled/evacuated by the spleen. The upadhatus of rakta are blood vessels and tendons. The mala is the pitta dosha itself.

If the pulse reader experiences imbalanced pitta qualities anywhere in the pulse, but especially expressed in the rakta dhatu crest, it could mean that its mala, pitta, is too high in the body overall, creating any condition associated with pitta. The pulse reader may also inquire about the state of the blood vessels in general, and symptoms such as inflamed tendons. Since the mala may be too high, the pulse reader should pay special attention to the organ of creation, the liver, and the organ of evacuation, the spleen. Many skin issues arise from excess pitta in the rakta dhatu due to issues related with the liver's ability to filter the blood.

If the pulse reader experiences imbalanced kapha qualities in the rakta dhatu pulse it could mean that the blood is too viscous or clotting too frequently. This could lead to conditions such as hypertension, diabetes, strokes etc. The pulse reader can inquire about the state of the upadhatus, which may indicate hyperflexible joints, swelling around the tendons, or blockages in blood vessels.

The mala, pitta, may be contaminated by ama leading to a variety of pitta-kapha related issues.

If the pulse reader experiences imbalanced vata qualities in the rakta dhatu pulse it could mean that the blood is too thin due to lack of production of the dhatu, there is improper clotting, or there are deformities in the red blood cells. This could lead to a myriad of conditions including anemia, vata rakta (arthritis), low blood pressure, etc. The pulse reader may also inquire about the state of the upadhatus which may indicate varicose veins or brittle or weak tendons. Brittle or weak tendons can result in strain or impaired movement anywhere muscle attaches to bone. For example, the tendons that move the eyes.

MAMSA DHATU

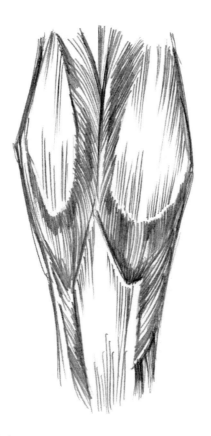

Image 40 - Mamsa Dhatu

Mamsa dhatu is the constituent that contributes largely to the creation of muscle tissue and functional membranes. Most organs are mainly comprised of varieties of mamsa dhatu. Mamsa dhatu is created primarily through muscle bundles themselves. After being initially created in the womb through the mother's dhatus, the muscle bundles become generators of the very tissue they are created from. Mamsa dhatu is evacuated by first becoming skin, and then as dead skin, though mamsa can be nourished via the skin as well. The upadhatus are skin, ligaments and a fatty membrane substance with the consistency of lard. The malas are dead skin cells and any kind of waxy substance expelled by the external orifices. For example, ear wax. Muscles are commonly thought of as a combination of mamsa and meda dhatu.

If the pulse reader experiences imbalanced vata qualities in the mamsa dhatu pulse it could mean that the muscle tissue is disproportionately sparse, weak or likely to incur injury. Organs can become displaced due to lack of integrity of membrane tissue, or constipation can occur because of a weakening of the colon tissues. Breathing issues can occur due to a lack of strength in the diaphragm and supportive muscles involved in respiration. The cardiac muscle may weaken resulting in low blood pressure. Membranes can, on a cellular level, become thin and impaired. Upon examining the upadhatus, the pulse reader may find thinning of the skin, excess dry, dead skin, cysts, stiffness in joints due to vata aggravated ligaments afflicted with excess dryness, or looseness in the joints due to lack of production of ligament tissue in later stages. The malas will be scanty or exceedingly dry.

If the pulse reader experiences imbalanced pitta qualities in the mamsa dhatu pulse, it could mean that the muscle tissue is too acidic. This is a primary cause for excessive inflammation in the body which leads to reduced overall regenerative capacity. Organ functions can become impaired under the influence of excess pitta, as the membranes themselves start to breakdown due to their exposure to hyperacidity. Upon examining the upadhatus the pulse reader may find a plethora of skin issues from rashes to acne to skin abscesses. Ligaments can become inflamed and compromise the function of joints and impair movement. The malas will be excessively odorous or abnormally colored.

If the pulse reader experiences imbalanced kapha qualities in the mamsa dhatu pulse, it could mean that the muscle tissue is too thick, dense, or overgrown or that growths are occurring in abnormal locations. This includes warts, tumors, cysts, polyps etc. The membranes and muscles may grow in a disproportionate manner, impairing movement and function. The skin may become excessively thick or become itchy. The ligaments may become disproportionate in relation to the bones and muscles, creating lack of stability in the individual's frame. The malas will be produced in too much abundance. In this case, the ears are most affected by the overproduction of earwax potentially clogging the ear canal.

MEDA DHATU

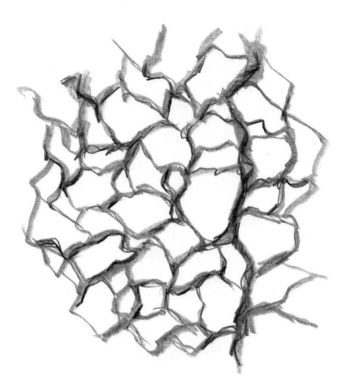

Image 41 - Meda Dhatu

Meda dhatu is the constituent that contributes largely to the creation of muscle tissue and adipose tissue. It is responsible for almost all lubrication in the body. Together, mamsa and meda create snayu, which is a muscle group. The mamsa dhatu creates the major structures of the muscle group and the meda dhatu creates the elasticity and fluidity of the muscle group. Fat is a storage house of meda, to be used as needed by the body. Meda is primarily created by omentum and evacuated primarily through the kidneys and sweat glands. The upadhatu of meda is muscle fiber and the mala is sweat.

If the pulse reader experiences imbalanced vata qualities in the meda dhatu pulse, it could mean that the rogi is experiencing some form of emaciation beyond that of healthy reduction of fat tissue. It could also mean that the body is not sufficiently lubricated, leading to a wide variety of issues throughout all the dhatus and organs. The upadhatu, muscles, may become weak, rigid and tight. Sweat as the mala may become sparse which can secondarily lead to issues with purifying the lymphatic fluids and skin.

If the pulse reader experiences imbalanced pitta qualities in the meda dhatu pulse, it could mean that the lubricants of the body are too acidic, causing widespread irritation to the other dhatus and organs by which the body responds with inflammation. Since the omentum and kidneys are the primary sites of meda dhatu, the intestines and kidneys may become more inflamed than other organs. The muscles, despite maintaining elasticity and strength, may produce too much lactic acid causing fatigue quickly. The sweat can become hyper acidic contributing to lymphatic issues and skin irritations.

If the pulse reader experiences imbalanced kapha qualities in the meda dhatu pulse, it could mean that the lubricants of the body are overproduced, causing the body to create more storage in the form of fat. This fat can cause weight gain but can also build up around the organs impairing their function. It can suppress the dhatu agnis as excess adipose tissue and lubricants clog channels, obstructing both pitta and vata. Muscles can become overgrown, develop lipomas, or become hyper elastic due to the disproportionate amount of meda to mamsa. Hernias can form due to the lack of fortitude of the abdominal wall. The sweat and lymphatic fluids may become profuse and contain high amounts of ama.

ASTHI DHATU

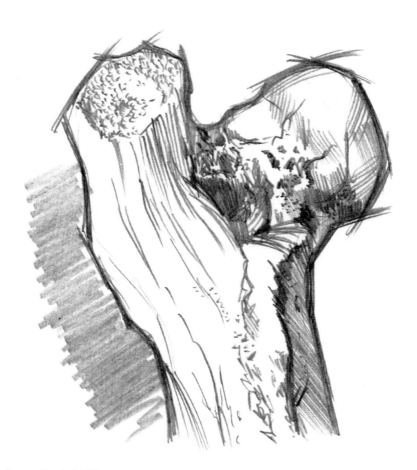

Image 42 - Asthi Dhatu

Asthi dhatu is the constituent that creates bone tissue, including cartilage. Bones are porous and play a crucial role in regulating the flow of vata through the body. They are extremely resistant to degeneration caused by the qualities associated with vata, in particular dryness. The primary site of origin is via the meda dhatu and the pelvic girdle. The primary site of evacuation is the colon. The upadhatus of asthi are teeth and the malas are hair and nails.

If the pulse reader experiences imbalanced vata qualities in the asthi dhatu pulse, it could mean that the rogi is suffering from osteoporosis, excessive popping and cracking in the joints or degenerative joint conditions such as arthritis. This can be caused by insubstantial bone production or insubstantial cartilage production. The upadhatus, teeth, may develop cavities, rough and ridged edges, or looseness within the gums due to the degradation of the roots of the teeth. The hair may become dry and brittle and an increase in hair loss may occur. The hair can also become patchy and slow to grow. The nails can become rough, feeble, tear easily and develop ridges or indentations.

Due to the nature of asthi dhatu, it is fairly resistant to the effects of pitta. The effects of pitta are best observed in the upadhatus and malas. If the pulse reader experiences imbalanced pitta qualities in the asthi dhatu pulse, it could mean that the rogi is experiencing sores in the mouth or abscesses in the teeth. It also increases the likelihood of cavities and gum infections. Large swaths of seemingly healthy hair may fall out due to excess heat traveling through the follicles, dilating the openings and weakening the hair roots. The nails may turn yellow and become susceptible to infections, including fungal infections.

If the pulse reader experiences imbalanced kapha qualities in the asthi dhatu pulse, it could mean that the rogi is suffering from bunions, bone spurs, significant deformity in bone structures or, in more advanced situations, bone tumors. The teeth may grow to be too large, crowding the mouth and creating dental issues. The hair may either grow excessively across the entire body, or the rogi may experience alopecia due to clogged follicles. The nails may develop white patches indicative of mineral deficiency caused by excess production of the malas.

MAJJA DHATU

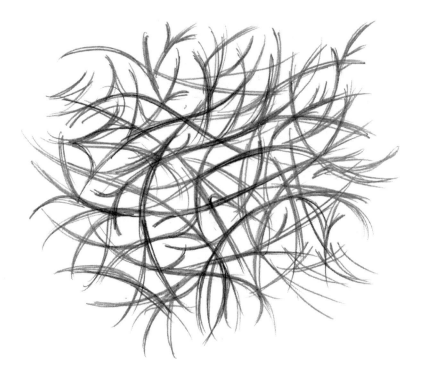

Image 43 - Majja Dhatu

Majja dhatu is a more refined form of meda dhatu that produces both bone marrow and cerebrospinal fluid. It is highly unctuous and liquid in nature. It is a storehouse of vital nutrition for the entire system. Majja dhatu is a primary constituent of nerve tissue, white brain matter and grey brain matter. A significant amount of the eye tissue is also comprised by majja dhatu. Every other dhatu in the body is innervated in some way by nerve tissue, and thus by majja dhatu. The primary sites of production are the bones and joints. The primary sites of evacuation are the kidneys. It is one of the most highly refined essences in the body and as such, it has no upadhatu. It produces very little of its mala, which partly contributes to the oily substance that nourishes hair and the discharge that emerges from the inside corners of the eyes.

An extremely large amount of interbody communication transfers through the majja dhatu in the form of nerves.

If the pulse reader experiences imbalanced vata qualities in the majja dhatu pulse, it may mean that the rogi is producing an insufficient amount of bone marrow, suffering from a wide variety of neurological problems, experiencing spasms, trembling, numbness, tingling, weakness, insomnia etc. There could be a lack of motor coordination. The eyes may become dry or malnourished. Brain activity may become either hyperactive or, less frequently, hypoactive. The rogi may feel constantly threatened, anxious, panicked, extremely sensitive or suffer from attention and focus disorders. Irregular heart palpitations may occur. In advanced cases it can indicate Parkinson's, various degrees of insanity, or dementia. The discharge from the eyes will likely not be present at all.

If the pulse reader experiences imbalanced pitta qualities in the majja dhatu pulse, it may mean that the rogi is suffering from pain in the form of burning, tearing or stabbing. The eyes are extremely sensitive to excess heat and may become red, irritated, or easily infected. It can also cause distortions in the shape of the pupil. The rogi may feel constantly irritated or angry without any apparent cause. Fevers can set in regardless of presence of viral or bacterial infections. The heart rate may increase excessively during activity. The intellect may become hyperactive when sadhaka pitta is excessively stimulated. In more advanced cases it can indicate Alzheimer's or multiple sclerosis. The discharge from the eyes may become infected, odorous or excessively sharp.

If the pulse reader experiences imbalanced kapha qualities in the majja dhatu pulse, it may indicate pain in the form of dullness, achiness or numbness due to blocked channels. The eyes can develop cataracts or glaucoma. Motor responses and reaction times could be delayed. The rogi may feel sluggish, intellectually dull, blank, depressed or excessively lethargic. The heart rate may become excessively slow. In more advanced cases there could be increased brain pressure, hydrocephalus, or nerve tumors including brain tumors. When combined with specific vata influences it could indicate autism.

SHURKA/ARTHAVA DHATU

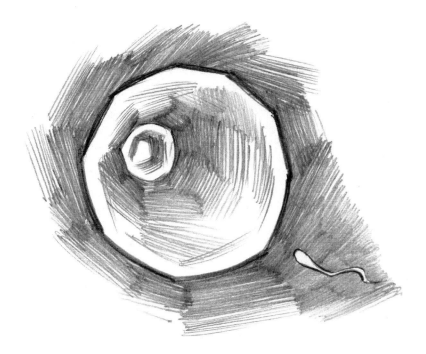

Image 44 - Shukra and Arthava Dhatus

The shukra dhatu comprises the reproductive fluids and tissues such as semen, sperm and ovum. It is accompanied by arthava in women only, which is not a dhatu in and of itself but commonly referred to as one. Shukra is produced and then circulated throughout every cell of the entire body. This allows for cellular reproduction. Both men and women have shukra dhatu which creates the channels related to pregnancy and menstrual flow. In men, the primary site of production is the testicles and in women the primary site of the production of shukra is breast tissue. The primary sites of production of arthava are the uterus and ovaries. The primary site of evacuation in men is the penis and in women the vaginal canal. Due to their highly refined natures, there are no upadhatus or malas. It is important to remember that menstrual fluids are the mala of rasa and not arthava.

Shukra pervades the entire body and its balance is vital to maintaining the prakruti. This is why balanced sexual activity is considered one of the three pillars of health next to sleep and ahara (food, water, air, and sense perceptions).

The shukra/arthava crest is felt under all three fingertips because it is so pervading in the body. The pulse reader should pay attention to which fingertips have active crests. If crests are present on two or three of the fingertips, then it signifies a very high degree of shukra/arthava activity. This could be an indication of the intensity of an imbalance. However, it could also indicate pregnancy, menstruation or ovulation which are not imbalances in and of themselves.

If the pulse reader experiences imbalanced vata qualities in the shukra/arthava dhatu pulse, then it could mean a depletion of the related tissues. This is not limited to semen, sperm and ovum but can cause depletion throughout the entire system influencing the generation of any of the dhatus. In the sexual realm, the rogi may be suffering from low libido, premature ejaculation, early onset menopause, low sperm count, scanty production of semen or sperm, erratic sperm motility, vaginal dryness, polycystic ovaries or difficulty maintaining erection. Excess vata in the arthava can cause difficulties with implantation of the fetus and miscarriages. The rogi may be adverse to, or anxious around sexual activity altogether. Outside of the sexual realm the rogi may feel discontent, uninspired, fatigued, anxious or fearful.

If the pulse reader experiences imbalanced pitta qualities in the shukra/arthava dhatu pulse, then the rogi may be suffering from an inflamed prostate due to hyper acidic semen, inflamed testicles, an inflamed vaginal canal, or imbalances in the acidity levels inside the vagina leading to yeast infections, pelvic inflammatory disease, and urinary tract infections in women and less commonly in men. The rogi may have too high of a libido or become too sexually aggressive. The pulse reader should inquire about a history of sexually transmitted diseases if she or he experiences imbalanced pitta qualities in the shukra/arthava pulse as the body responds to them primarily through a pitta driven response. Outside of the sexual realm the rogi may feel angry, irritable, violent or desirous of taking extreme risks.

If the pulse reader experiences imbalanced kapha qualities in the shukra/arthava dhatu pulse, then the rogi may be suffering from testicular swelling, have a hydrocele, vaginal swelling, cysts, polyps, or tumors. The sperm motility can become sluggish. In men, ejaculation may not occur even when desired. Menopause may be delayed. Kapha imbalances can also indicate yeast infections in women. The rogi may experience low libido, not from the lack of production of shukra but from a lack of enthusiasm for and enjoyment of sexual activity. Outside of the sexual realm the rogi may feel depressed, unmotivated, heavy and congested.

THE DHATUS, THEIR SITES OF ORIGIN, ELIMINATION, UPADHATUS & MALAS

DHATU	ORIGIN	ELIMINATION	UPADHATU	MALA
RASA	HEART & BLOOD VESSELS	SKIN, KIDNEYS, FECES	MENSTRUAL FLUIDS, BREAST MILK	KAPHA
RAKTA	LIVER	SPLEEN	BLOOD VESSELS & TENDONS	PITTA
MAMSA	MUSCLE BUNDLES	DEAD SKIN	SKIN, LIGAMENTS, MUSCLE FIBERS	WAXY DISCHARGE INCLUDING EARWAX
MEDA	OMENTUM & KIDNEYS	KIDNEYS	LUBRICATION FLUIDS	SWEAT
ASTHI	PELVIC GIRDLE	VIA MEDA DHATU	TEETH	HAIR & NAILS
MAJJA	LARGE BONES	JOINTS & KIDNEYS	NONE	UNCTUOUS COATINGS FOUND ON OTHER FORMS OF DISCHARGE
SHUKRA	BREASTS & SCROTUM	PENIS & VAGINA	NONE	NONE
ARTHAVA	UTERUS & OVERIES	VAGINA	NONE	NONE

A NOTE ON OJAS

Ojas is the most refined substance in the body and is created through the contributions of all the dhatus acting in harmony. It is the fuel by which the immune system operates and creates the body's overall resilience to internal and external destabilizing influences. It is not directly read on the fifth layer of the pulse but assessing the health

87

of all the dhatus is crucial in the assessment of ojas. Its status is read directly on the fourth layer of the pulse instead.

EXAMPLE OF A FIFTH LAYER PULSE

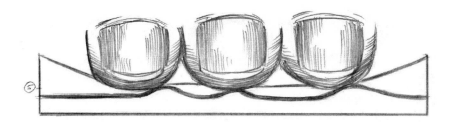

Image 45 - Example of a Fifth Layer Pulse

The crests are expressing themselves via the rakta dhatu on the ring fingertip, shukra dhatu on the middle fingertip and majja dhatu on the index fingertip. This information alone communicates that these three dhatus are active in the body. It is not always the case that a crest will be felt under each fingertip, or that one of the crests may be much more prominent than the others.

If, for instance, the crest under all three fingertips is expressing primarily vata qualities the pulse reader should pay attention to deep seated depletion in the body as two of the deepest dhatus, majja and shukra, are showing signs of vata imbalance. Rakta, shukra and majja are all comprised primarily of jala, the water element, so a pulse such as the above could indicate an imbalance as simple as dehydration.

If, for instance, the crest under all three fingertips is expressing primarily pitta qualities, the pulse reader should pay attention to blood related issues caused by hyper acidity that have become deep seated. Gout being one example. The rogi may also be experiencing symptoms associated with excess pitta in the shukra or arthava dhatus.

If, for instance, the crest under all three fingertips is expressing primarily kapha qualities, the pulse reader should pay attention to deep seated ama formation affecting cellular reproduction due to the shukra involvement. The entire body may ache. In advanced cases this type of pulse signature could be an indication of malignant tumor growth. If the entirety of the pulse is very feeble, including the seventh layer pulse, the pulse reader should become more alert to this possibility. The excessive reproduction of cells creates the malignant component of the pathology. The rakta dhatu circulates ama throughout the body continuously creating an environment in which the malignant cells can obtain nutrition. The involvement of majja confirms the depth of penetration the ama has achieved and negatively affects the body's ability to communicate with itself to activate the immune system appropriately.

Frequently, the pulse expresses qualities corresponding to multiple doshas under different fingertips. In such situations, the pulse reader must discern which qualities are the most prominent and most related to the other layers of the pulse. The possibilities are immense

---

COMMON MISTAKE

In many individuals the index fingertip pulse is the clearest and easiest to read. As such, it can appear more prominent than the pulses on the middle and ring fingertips. When reading the fifth layer of the pulse it is common to pick up on asthi and majja dhatus first. The pulse reader should not let this distract him or her from deeply concentrating on the other fingertips.

CHAPTER NINE

READING THE VITAL ORGANS IN THE PULSE LAYERS ONE AND SEVEN

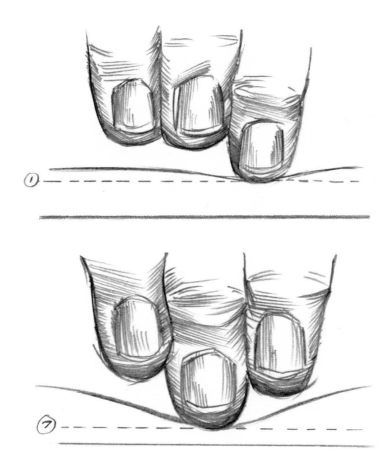

Image 46 - Reading the Organ Pulses

The vital organs are read on the first and seventh layers of the pulse using only one fingertip at a time. The other two fingertips may be removed from the skin altogether or gently touch the skin not perceiving even the first layer of the pulse. Three locations are read on each fingertip in the same manner as the seventh, fifth and first layers. The pulse reader must read both the right and left radial arteries individually to ascertain information from all of the vital organs.

There are two important methods of practice when reading the vital organs. The first, as always, is to experience the qualities expressed by the crest. In general, a healthy organ will express similar qualities as the overall feeling found in the prakruti layer. The second is to compare the organ pulse on the first layer with the organ pulse on the seventh layer associated with the same finger. If one or the other is much weaker or completely absent, then it is an indication suggesting that the corresponding organ is imbalanced or functioning under stress. If both organs associated with one finger feel weak compared to the organs associated with the other fingers, then it suggests that both organs associated with that finger are imbalanced or operating under stress. What this leads the pulse reader to is the practice of checking multiple organs under multiple fingers to get a general baseline of the strength of each organ before honing-in on information expressed by individual organ pulses.

Reading the seventh layer of the pulse for prakruti or the first layer of the pulse for vikruti is not the same as reading an organ on the seventh layer or the first layer. In reading the prakruti or vikruti pulse all three fingertips are compressing the radial artery. In reading an organ pulse only one finger is compressing that portion of the radial artery. This prompts the pulse to express itself differently as the flow of blood through the artery is altered in an altogether different manner.

The vital organs are composed of the dhatus and home to the most vital functions of the body to take place. As such, they are inextricably intertwined with the subdoshas. While not all of the organs are strictly necessary to sustain life, the vikruti becomes severely disturbed by the malfunction or absence of any of them. For example, missing gallbladder creates impaired digestive function. A non-functional kidney greatly reduces the body's ability to filter fluids.

THE PULSE AND CORRESPONDING ORGAN LOCATIONS

SIDE	LEFT RADIAL ARTERY		RIGHT RADIAL ARTERY	
FINGER	FIRST LAYER	SEVENTH LAYER	FIRST LAYER	SEVENTH LAYER
INDEX	SMALL INTESTINE	HEART	COLON	LUNGS
MIDDLE	STOMACH	SPLEEN & PANCREAS	GALLBLADDER	LIVER
RING	BLADDER	KIDNEYS	PERICARDIUM	CIRCULATION

LEFT RADIAL ARTERY ORGANS

FIRST LAYER – INDEX FINGER – THE SMALL INTESTINE AND DUODENUM

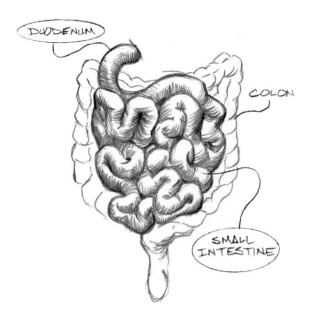

Image 47 - Small Intestine and Duodenum

The small intestine is longer, but smaller in diameter than the large intestine. Its primary function is to slowly move nourishment through its tract via peristalsis while samana vata separates nourishment from waste to be converted to rasa dhatu and then disseminated to the other organs and dhatus. It ultimately transitions into the large intestine, which is the colon.

The duodenum is the "C" shaped portion of the small intestine that attaches directly to the bottom of the stomach. The duodenum is one of the seats of the primary agni in the body, jathar agni. Food and liquids are released from the stomach into the duodenum where they are mixed with a variety of digestive enzymes, such as insulin from the pancreas, and bile from the liver and gallbladder. The substance created from this mixture of food, bile and other digestive enzymes is called chyme.

If the functions of the small intestine are impaired, especially the duodenum, then all of the agnis in the body will eventually become impaired.

The pulse reader should pay special attention to imbalances expressed by the small intestine pulse in relationship with samana vata, pachaka pitta, kledaka kapha and bodhaka kapha.

Samana vata is responsible for moving chyme through the small intestines. Too fast and the body cannot absorb nourishment quickly enough. Too slow and ama can form clogging the channels of transfer. This can be a cause of an inflammatory intestinal disorder as the immune system will create inflammation in an attempt to restore the channels to their proper function.

Pachaka pitta resides primarily in the stomach but is released into the duodenum along with ingested food and liquid. The duodenum does not have as much protective lining as the stomach in the form of kledaka kapha and is more susceptible to damage from hyper-acidity. If pachaka pitta is too weak, then the mixture of digestives needed to produce chyme will not be potent enough, creating indigestion and ama.

Kledaka kapha resides primarily in the stomach as a protective lining. If too much sluffs off and is released into the duodenum it can weaken the jathar agni and create indigestion. In more advanced stages this begins the pathology of type two diabetes. Kledaka kapha enters the duodenum, is not fully digested and then enters the remaining intestines and gets absorbed into the bloodstream, increasing blood sugar and eventually clogging the kidneys. Bodhaka kapha resides primarily in the mouth but also contributes to the digestive mixtures in the stomach and small intestine. It labels food via taste, informing the body of which digestive enzymes to release.

SEVENTH LAYER – INDEX FINGER – THE HEART

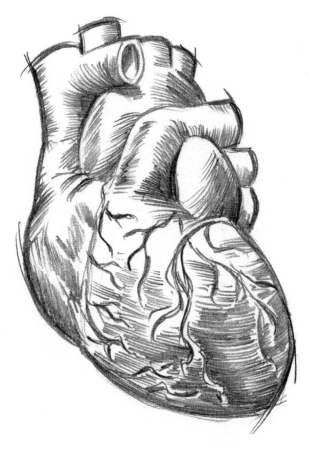

Image 48 - Heart

The primary function of the heart is to maintain balanced circulation by pumping blood. To stop there would be to gravely oversimplify its significance. It is a highly sophisticated organ that acts as the center to multiple subdoshic functions. It receives and responds to a tremendous amount of information from the nervous system on a moment to moment basis. It is also crucial to the digestive process. It assesses the quality of the blood by measuring the flavor of blood via built-in bitter taste receptors. The same type found on the tongue. It alters its own function in response, which in turn alters the function of every other organ in the body.

Ayurvedic wisdom considers the heart as the seat of the mind. Heart related imbalances greatly affect an individual's perceptual experiences via the mind.

The pulse reader should pay special attention to imbalances expressed by the heart pulse in relationship with prana vata, udana vata, vyana vata, apana vata, sadhaka pitta, and kapha in general, especially avalambaka kapha.

All of the subdoshas of vata directly affect the function of the heart with the exception of samana, which still indirectly affects heart function via digestion. Prana vata and vyana vata are seated in the heart so the proper function of the heart is vital to their function and vice versa. Udana vata, while not seated in the heart, is very sensitive to its function. Respiration and heart rate go together part and parcel. Apana vata is also not seated in the heart but heavily influences and is influenced by prana. Issues with elimination are among the primary causes of heart imbalances, especially those related to heart rate and rhythm.

Sadhaka pitta is seated in the heart. This makes the heart, and not the brain the primary organ of intelligence. Intelligence here does not simply mean common human intellect. Rather it refers to the intelligence within each cell of the body. Heart issues severely impact brain function but the reverse is not always true. Sadhaka pitta also plays an important role in the brain but its primary function originates in the heart.

95

Kapha is present in the blood and thus circulates through the heart. Too much can clog the arteries and veins causing restricted blood flow, high blood pressure or, in advanced cases, heart attack. Too little and the blood becomes too thin. The heart then has to work harder to maintain balanced circulation. Avalambaka kapha forms the fluid inside the pericardium which envelops and protects the heart. Depletion of avalambaka kapha can leave the heart vulnerable to damage. Excess avalambaka kapha can restrict the heart's function via compression caused by swelling.

The pulse reader must always remember that the seat of the mind is in the heart not the brain. The mind can pervade any part of the body but its "home" is in the heart. When an individual focuses her or his awareness and intention in the heart then it gives the opportunity to the mind to reside on its natural throne. Remember that prana vata, vyana vata, and sadhaka pitta are also seated in the heart. A distressed heart pulse can convey valuable information about the status of the rogi's mind.

FIRST LAYER – MIDDLE FINGER – THE STOMACH

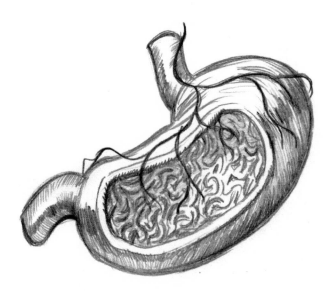

Image 49 - Stomach Innervated by the Vagus Nerve

The primary function of the stomach is to digest whole foods and liquids. It is both extremely tough and elastic, capable of handling high levels of acidity and changing size to accommodate various amounts of food. The stomach is home to jathar agni. The majority of gross digestion occurs in both the stomach and small intestine, specifically in the duodenum.

The pulse reader should pay special attention to imbalances expressed by the stomach pulse in relationship with prana vata, samana vata, pachaka pitta, kledaka kapha and bodhaka kapha.

All of the vata subdoshas play a role in stomach function but prana vata and samana vata play the most significant roles. Prana vata governs the movement of food into the stomach. Samana vata regulates how much and when pachaka pitta is released in concord with the activity of prana while eating. Samana vata then orchestrates the movement of the nutritional mixture into the duodenum. If samana vata is out of balance, then the stomach does not release the appropriate amount of hydrochloric acid. Food either does not get broken down well enough, resulting in ama, or gets broken down too much, destroying the food's nutritional value.

The stomach is the seat of pachaka pitta. The stomach walls secrete a form of hydrochloric acid that cooks foods and liquids breaking them down into smaller components. It also kills most types of harmful viruses, bacteria and parasites. If pachaka pitta is too potent, the acid can burn through the protective lining of the stomach and cause damage to the organ tissues. This, in time, can form ulcers. If pachaka pitta is too weak then food will not break down properly, leading to the creation of ama. It also makes the body susceptible to food borne bacteria and parasites. If pachaka pitta is produced in too much quantity, but not necessarily too potent, then reflux may occur.

The stomach is the seat of kledaka kapha. Kledaka kapha forms protective linings of the stomach. The balance between kledaka kapha and pachaka pitta is crucial to the functioning of the entire body. They keep each other in check. Too little kledaka kapha and pachaka pitta cannot be contained. Too much kledaka kapha results in a sluffing effect that leads to indigestion, ama creation and the beginnings of clogged channels throughout the body, especially the heart, liver and kidneys. The digestion of food begins with bodhaka kapha in the mouth. Weak bodhaka kapha hampers the effectiveness of the stomach while excessively potent bodhaka kapha contributes to hyperacidity in the stomach. Excessive bodhaka kapha can also dilute stomach acid to a degree.

SEVENTH LAYER – MIDDLE FINGER – SPLEEN AND PANCREAS

THE SPLEEN

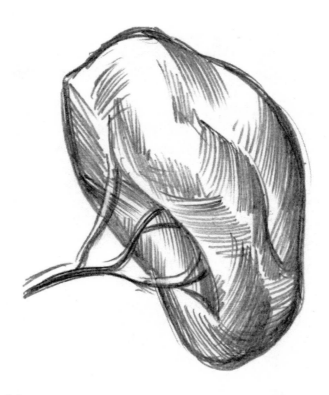

Image 50 - Spleen

The spleen is located to the left of the stomach. Its primary function is to remove damaged, dead, malformed and poorly functioning red blood cells from circulation. It does so with a pulp-like filtration structure. It preserves important nourishment from the blood that can be reused by healthy blood cells.

The pulse reader should pay special attention to imbalances expressed by the spleen pulse in relationship with vyana vata, pachaka pitta and avalambaka kapha.

The spleen is quite relevant to the process of the circulation of blood. Hence, vyana vata is most important to its function. Blood continuously flows through the spleen, subject to its filtration. If vyana vata is too strong then the filtration of blood does not occur sufficiently enough. Too weak and the filtration process stagnates.

Pachaka pitta deals with the breakdown of red blood cells tagged for elimination. If pachaka pitta is too strong in the spleen, then it will start to damage the organ itself. If it is too weak then red blood cells will not be destroyed properly, resulting in the formation of a type of blood-based ama. If this goes on for too long the spleen can become enlarged.

Avalambaka kapha forms the protective linings of the spleen. The spleen generates a great deal of heat due to the prominent presence of pachaka pitta. It is the role of avalambaka kapha to contain this heat properly. If avalambaka kapha is too weak, then the organ itself can get damaged even if pachaka pitta is not too high. If avalambaka kapha is too prominent, it can cause swelling in the spleen, altering its function.

THE PANCREAS

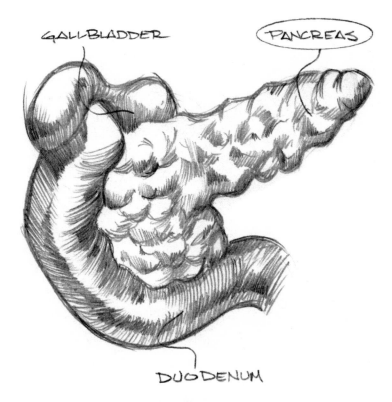

Image 51 - Pancreas

The pancreas is located primarily behind the stomach and extends to the left towards the spleen. Its primary function is to produce pancreatic enzymes and hormones to aid in the digestion of fat, sugar and starch. Insulin is the most renown of these which is critical in the digestion of glucose.

The pulse reader should pay special attention to imbalances expressed by the pancreas pulse in relationship with samana vata, apana vata, pachaka pitta and kledaka kapha.

Similar to the stomach, samana vata governs the quantity and timing of the release of the pancreas' digestive fluids. The actual secretion of these fluids into the duodenum is governed by apana vata. If these two forces are not in balance with each other then the secretion will not happen in harmony with the activities in the stomach and small intestine leading to imbalanced digestion.

Pachaka pitta is responsible for the generation of the appropriate mixture of digestive enzymes and hormones within the pancreas. However, unlike the stomach, this mixture is less acidic. If pachaka pitta is imbalanced in the pancreas then the digestive mixture will be inappropriate in relation to the type and quantity of food consumed and the small intestine will be hampered in its functions.

Kledaka kapha resides in the stomach. However, it combines with food particles to protect them from excess exposure to pachaka pitta. A portion of kledaka kapha combines with glucose and gets released into the duodenum along with the food it protects. The proper digestion of kledaka kapha in the duodenum is dependent on insulin, which is created by the pancreas alone.

FIRST LAYER – RING FINGER – THE BLADDER

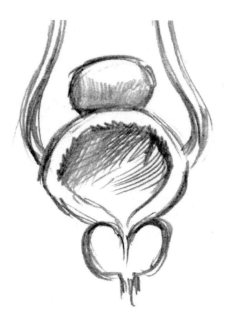

Image 52 - Bladder

The bladder is considered one of the primary abodes of lifeforce in the body. Its primary function is to store and evacuate urine. It is highly elastic holding potentially large volumes of liquid before requiring release.

The pulse reader should pay special attention to imbalances expressed by the bladder pulse in relationship with apana vata, pitta in general, ranjaka pitta, and kapha in general.

The bladder is one of the seats of apana vata along with the colon as it is a major site of evacuation of one of the primary malas. Withholding the natural urges, including urination, is one of the foremost contributors to the progression of imbalances. An inability to urinate, or unwillingness to urinate disturbs the flow of apana vata, which then begins to obstruct the flow of all the other subdoshas of vata. Excessive urination can be a sign of hyperactive apana vata, which will result in depletion and weakness throughout the body.

Unused pitta dosha is evacuated through the bladder via urine. If bladder function becomes impaired, then pitta cannot be evacuated properly and builds up throughout the body.

Ranjaka pitta is responsible for the color of urine. In excess the urine becomes dark yellow. When balanced the urine is primarily clear with a yellow tint. Completely clear urine can be a sign of weak ranjaka pitta and its associated functions.

If kapha is too abundant the body releases an inappropriate amount of water to aid the kidneys in filtration. This is then released through the bladder as a diluted form of urine. It is also one of the causes of excessive urination. This urine often has a sweet odor due to the undigested kapha it contains. If kledaka kapha is not abundant enough it could result in scanty urination. This indicates insufficient hydration or improper circulation of liquids throughout the body, especially if there is swelling in other regions.

SEVENTH LAYER – RING FINGER – THE KIDNEYS

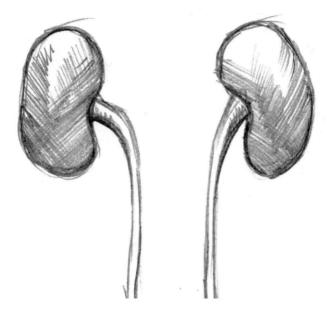

Image 53 - Kidneys

The kidneys are located above the waistline protected by the ribs. Their primary function is to filter blood and liquids for either reassimilation or evacuation. If the kidneys are functioning properly, the reassimilated liquids return with balanced mineral content. Poorly functioning kidneys return liquid to the body full of ama that should have been filtered and evacuated. Both pitta and kapha share the water element in their basic makeup. The kidneys take on a vital role of maintaining the purity of pitta and kapha throughout the entire body. Both excess pitta and kapha are evacuated by balanced kidney function. The kidneys are also the primary evacuation site of meda and majja dhatu, two of the most unctuous dhatus. The adrenal glands (not depicted) rest on top of each kidney and are intimately connected with kidney activity.

The pulse reader should pay special attention to imbalances expressed by the kidney pulse in relationship with apana vata, vyana vata, pitta in general, ranjaka pitta, and kapha in general.

Apana vata influences the rate and intensity with which fluids flow through the kidneys. Too strong and proper filtration cannot occur. Too weak and toxicity can build up in kidney tissues creating issues ranging from kidney stones to renal failure. Lower back pain due to kidney imbalances can be caused by imbalanced apana vata as well.

The kidneys filter pitta from the blood and pass it through to the bladder to be evacuated. Excess pitta can damage the kidney tissue. Too little indicates weak agni, and the presence of ama which will clog the kidney channels. Ranjaka pitta gives urine its color. Imbalances expressed in both the ranjaka pitta pulse and the kidney pulse should prompt the pulse reader to inquire regarding the quality and quantity of the rogi's urine.

The kidneys are the primary filter for the jala element in the body, which is one of the elements that forms kapha. As such, the kidneys must manage the evacuation of excess kapha on a constant basis. The sticky nature of kapha can be a primary cause of kidney blockages if too abundant or if present in the form of ama.

RIGHT RADIAL ARTERY ORGANS

FIRST LAYER – INDEX FINGER – THE COLON

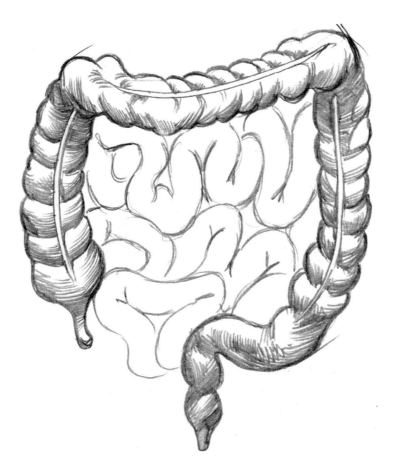

Image 54 - Colon

The colon is referred to in four sections. The ascending colon, the transverse colon, the descending colon and the sigmoid colon. The primary functions of the colon are to reabsorb liquids from the digestive process back into the bloodstream and prepare the remnants of the digestive process, namely feces, for elimination. The colon is the primary seat of the vata dosha and plays a vital role in any activity involving vata. This means every activity in the body in some way or another. Balance in the colon is imperative to sustaining balance in the body.

The pulse reader should pay special attention to imbalances expressed by the colon in relationship to all of the subdoshas of vata but especially apana vata and samana vata, pitta in general, ranjaka pitta, and kapha in general.

Apana vata is the primary subdosha that governs how well feces are eliminated. If it is too weak then constipation can occur. If it is too strong then feces cannot form fully, or water absorption does not happen properly, and diarrhea can occur. If apana vata is strong enough to eliminate but elimination cannot occur due to another factor, then apana reverses its flow and begins disturbing all of the other subdoshas of vata. Samana vata plays a large role in peristalsis. Too weak and constipation can occur, not because of weak apana vata but because of weak peristaltic action. The feces do not move through the colon at an adequate rate. The opposite is true in the form of diarrhea if samana vata is too strong.

Pitta is evacuated through the colon as the end product of bile contained within feces. Ranjaka pitta gives stool its color via the quantity and quality of bile released during the earlier stages of digestion. Bile is a yellow green color when released into the small intestine. Feces acquires its brown color primarily in the colon. Stool may keep its yellow or greenish color if the colon is not processing ranjaka pitta properly or too much ranjaka pitta is being created in the digestive process for the colon to properly handle.

Kapha is comprised mostly of the earth element and excess kapha is evacuated through the colon as stool. The nature of kapha in the body impacts the health of the colon greatly. If kapha is too sticky, then it adheres to the colon walls impairing the proper transfer of fluids to and from the bloodstream. If stool is too scanty then the force of vata accumulates in its seat potentially aggravating vata throughout the rest of the body.

SEVENTH LAYER – INDEX FINGER – THE LUNGS

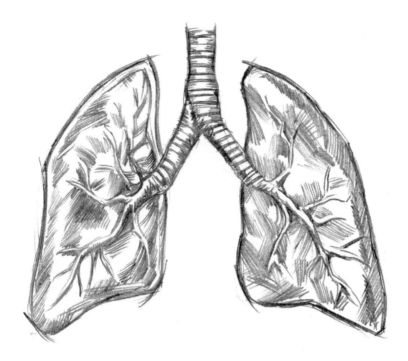

Image 55 - Lungs

The primary function of the lungs is to filter inhaled air so that the blood can collect oxygen, and then exhale carbon dioxide along with other metabolic wastes. The lungs play a major role in detoxifying the body, not just from what is in the external environment, but also clearing ama that has been metabolized within the body and needs to be evacuated. The lungs are the seat of udana vata and avalambaka kapha. Its movements are primarily regulated via the diaphragm which controls the expansion and contraction of the lungs changing the internal pressure balance. The movement of the lungs and diaphragm affects the heart. Faster lung and diaphragm movement increases heart rate and vice versa.

The pulse reader should pay special attention to imbalances expressed by the lungs in relationship to prana vata, udana vata, pitta in general and avalambaka kapha.

Inhalation via the lungs is the primary means by which the body receives prana from the environment. Imbalance in the lungs can result in an overall depletion of prana, affecting all functions, tissues and organs in the body. Too much prana flowing into the body at one time can cause mental disturbances ranging from minor to severe. The stability of the mind and heart rely on the vitality of the lungs. Udana vata governs the exhalation. Weak lungs, or impaired exhalation creates a major toxicity issue for the body. The breath-to-breath refreshment healthy lungs provide is compromised, not only by carbon dioxide but by other forms of ama build up in the bloodstream unable to be released via exhalation. Unable to expel these poisons, the remainder of the organs become impaired or begin to fail fairly rapidly.

Of the three doshas, pitta has the least prevalence in the lungs. However, the lungs are constantly exposed to pitta via the immense amount of blood that flows through them. If pitta is too potent in the bloodstream then the lung tissue easily become damaged making them susceptible to infections.

Avalambaka kapha forms the protective lining both inside and outside of the lung tissue. It ensures that the bronchial passages and alveoli are shielded from excess vata, pitta and ama. Damage to the lung tissue can aggravate avalambaka kapha, which also protects the heart. Avalambaka kapha is very sensitive to stress and emotionality. Hence, the lungs can experience deterioration from excess of either of these influences. Excess kapha of any form in the lungs creates conditions in which the blood has difficulty retrieving oxygen and expelling carbon dioxide and other metabolic wastes due to clogged passageways, of which the lungs have over one billion.

FIRST LAYER – MIDDLE FINGER – THE GALLBLADDER

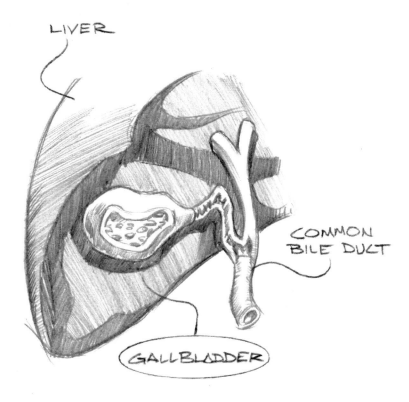

Image 56 - Gallbladder

The gallbladder is located on the right side of the body and rests against the underside of the liver. Its primary function is to assist with the storage and potency of the bile produced by the liver. It is an important organ for the digestion of all forms of fat and oil.

The pulse reader should pay special attention to imbalances expressed by the gallbladder in relationship to samana vata, apana vata, pachaka pitta and kapha in general.

Samana vata plays a similar role in the gallbladder as it does in the stomach and pancreas. It orchestrates the quantity and timing of release of stored bile into the digestive mixture contained within the duodenum. Apana vata governs the actual secretion of this bile into the common bile duct, shared by the gallbladder and liver, into the small intestine. If either samana vata or apana vata are imbalanced, then chyme will not be formed properly resulting in digestive disturbances.

Pachaka pitta is the primary subdosha responsible for the generation of bile. Bile receives its color from ranjaka pitta. If pachaka pitta is too strong then the gallbladder can become damaged and inflamed. If pachaka pitta is too weak then excess kapha can build up in the gallbladder contributing to the creation of gallstones.

Since the gallbladder's primary function is to assist the liver in the breakdown of fats and oils, its association with kapha is important. If kapha is expressing itself too prominently in the gallbladder then the gallbladder becomes overwhelmed and cannot assist the liver adequately. This then creates extra strain on the other digestive organs.

SEVENTH LAYER – MIDDLE FINGER – THE LIVER

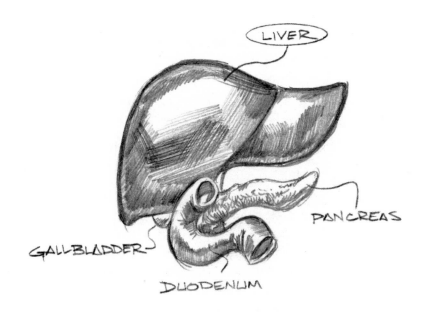

Image 57 - Liver

The liver is located on the right side of the body mostly under the ribcage. It is very close in proximity to the duodenum and pancreas. The liver has a vast variety of functions. It is one of the most industrious organs in the body. Some of its primary functions are to produce bile, to discern what should remain in the bloodstream and what should be removed, and to store minerals, chemicals and nutrition for later use. Blood flows through the liver from the intestines and stomach prior to reaching the heart. Thus, the liver plays an important role in protecting the heart from exposure to compromised blood.

The pulse reader should pay special attention to imbalances expressed by the liver in relationship to samana vata, apana vata, pitta in general and all of its subdoshas, and kapha in general.

Samana vata and apana vata function the same way for the liver as they do for the gallbladder, stomach and pancreas. Samana vata organizes the plethora of digestive fluids the liver generates as well as the timing of their release in accordance with the information relayed by the sense organs and stomach. Apana vata controls the actual secretion of the digestive fluids through the common bile duct into the duodenum. If there is an imbalance in either of these functions, then improper or incomplete digestion of food is guaranteed.

The liver is profoundly and intimately connected with the pitta dosha and all of its subdoshic activity. Pachaka pitta forms bile, the liver's primary digestive creation. The liver is the root organ of ranjaka pitta giving color to the blood, bile, urine and feces. While not directly connected to bhrajaka pitta, which resides in the skin, the liver must filter that which bhrajaka pitta cannot handle via transdermal digestion. Weaknesses in bhrajaka pitta affect the liver greatly. The liver manages the heat levels of the blood. Alochaka pitta and eye tissue is highly sensitive to the heat content in blood. Liver issues frequently manifest through the eyes. Lastly, sadhaka pitta generates the discernment the liver applies to all of the blood that flows through it from the stomach and small intestine, prior to reaching the heart and then the rest of the body. Liver issues can also affect sadhaka pitta's function, which can have an impact on the functions of the heart and brain.

As a primary filter of blood, the liver must discern what remains in the bloodstream and what must be evacuated. Kapha that has been deemed excess by the liver is removed through the excretion of bile into the small intestine and becomes part of the formation of feces. If kapha is too prominent in the body then the liver cannot filter all of it out and becomes toxified, impairing the liver's function. The blood becomes compromised and the organs further down the bloodstream begin accumulating ama.

FIRST LAYER – RING FINGER – THE PARICARDIUM

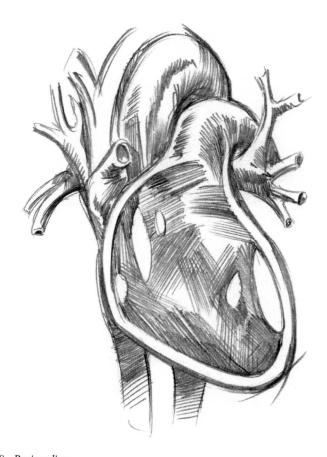

Image 58 - Pericardium

The pericardium envelops the heart and is primarily composed of avalambaka kapha. Its primary functions are to nourish and protect the heart. It does so by keeping the heart lubricated and shielded from impacts and unwanted substances.

The pulse reader should pay special attention to imbalances expressed by the pericardium in relationship to prana vata, vyana vata, sadhaka pitta, and avalambaka kapha.

Any subdosha of vata related to the heart will relate to the pericardium. The pericardium's role in accordance with the subdoshas of vata is to protect their proper functioning in the heart. If the pericardium is impaired, then the heart becomes vulnerable and the subdoshas of vata become more easily agitated.

Again, the pericardium's role in accordance with sadhaka pitta is to protect its proper functioning within the heart. Sadhaka pitta is highly sensitive to the condition of the pericardium as damage to the pericardium typically signals impending damage to the heart. Rogis with an imbalance in the pericardium often suffer from high levels of stress, emotionality and are easily triggered.

The pericardium is primarily composed of avalambaka kapha. If avalambaka kapha is too prominent, then the pericardium may become swollen, putting undue pressure on the heart. If avalambaka kapha is too weak, then the heart and its functions become too vulnerable and sensitive to the fluctuations in the internal and external environments.

SEVENTH LAYER – RING FINGER – THE CIRCULATORY SYSTEM

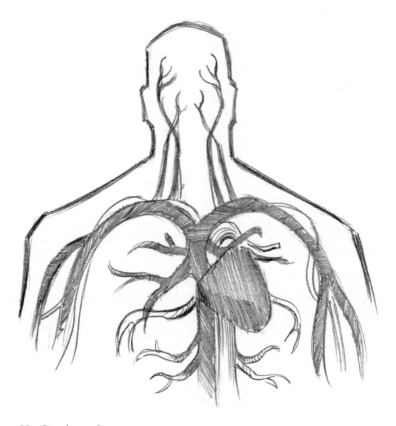

Image 59 - Circulatory System

The circulatory system pervades the entire body. It is not a vital organ but its function and stability as a whole can be experienced on the rogi's right side, seventh layer, ring finger pulse. The circulatory system moves much more than blood. It also mobilizes the entire lymphatic system. The circulation of the lymphatic system is dependent on the proper circulation of blood.

The primary function of circulation is to continuously provide the means to receive, distribute and dispose of all nourishment in all forms so that the agni, the core metabolic force, may remain in balance.

There is no specific subdosha the pulse reader should pay special attention to with the exceptions of prana vata and vyana vata. Every subdosha is influenced by the status of the circulatory system and is in some way dependent on the proper functioning of the circulatory system to move throughout the body.

If the vata dosha is too strong then the pressure circulation exerts on the tissues becomes too intense, creating stress damage over time. If the vata dosha is too weak then circulation becomes sluggish and the dhatus do not receive proper nourishment. If the pitta dosha is too strong then too much heat and acid circulate into every tissue and organ causing damage. If the pitta dosha is too weak then the circulatory system contracts and constricts, hampering its flow. If the kapha dosha is too prominent then the circulatory system can become clogged and blocked creating unnatural movements of vata as well as obstructive disorders. If kapha is too weak then the tissues involved in circulation become to brittle, unable to contain the pressure exerted by the force of vata.

IMPORTANT NOTES ON THE "MISSING" VITAL ORGANS

There is no individual pulse for two very prominent features of the body. The brain and the skin. There is a specific reason for their absence amongst the pantheon of vital organ pulses. Ayurvedically speaking, the brain is an extension of majja dhatu, organized primarily by prana vata, sadhaka pitta and tarpaka kapha. The pulse reader can assess the rogi's brain by synthesizing these pulse expressions.

The skin is the upadhatu of mamsa. It is highly sensitive to the activities of all the vata subdoshas and the primary realm of bhrajaka pitta. The skin is not simply a layer of protection but a sophisticated digestive system. Bhrajaka pitta is to the skin as pachaka pitta is to the stomach. The pulse reader can assess the quality of the skin by synthesizing information from the state of vata in general, bhrajaka pitta specifically, and the presence of ama in the system. High levels of ama dramatically influence the skin's ability to absorb nutrition and excrete waste in the forms of dead skin and sweat.

EXAMPLE OF A VITAL ORGAN PULSE

Detailed examples of reading the organ pulses are found in chapter sixteen.

COMMON MISTAKE

The pulse reader hyper focuses on a particular organ, especially one showing obvious signs of imbalance and manifesting symptoms. While it is of course important to address the immediate needs of a distressed organ, the zoom of the pulse reader's lens should be widened in the effort to discover what is creating the imbalance coming to a head within a specific organ.

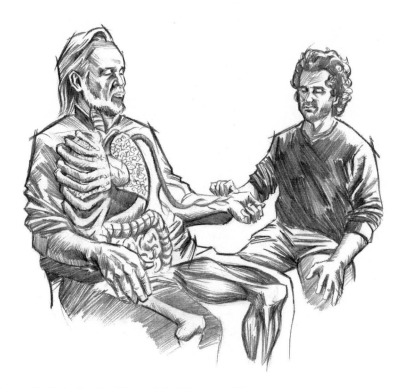

Image 60 - Pulse Reader "Seeing" the Dhatus and Organs

CHAPTER TEN

TENDENCIES TOWARDS SATTVA, RAJAS AND TAMAS THE SIXTH LAYER OF THE PULSE

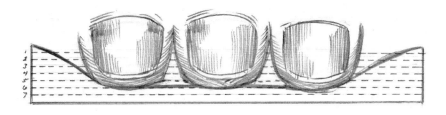

Image 61 - The Sixth Layer

The sixth layer of the pulse expresses an individual's inherent leanings towards sattva, rajas and tamas. Observing this layer of the pulse helps reveal the nature of an individual's mind. Sattva, rajas and tamas are the three mental gunas. They are the forces which the mind utilizes to perform its functions. Rajas and tamas have a pull of their own. The mind can become overly habitual in their use and, in a sense, become addicted.

Sattva in its essence is clear, balanced, neutrality. Rajas in its essence is activity. Tamas in its essence is inertia.

Sattva is the capacity that allows for the integrated use of both rajas and tamas in order to consciously create anything in the manifest world. An individual can never have "too much" sattva while it is possible to engage with too much rajas or too much tamas. A sattva-oriented mind can perceive the whole, the truth, both subtleties and the overt, and do so without reacting subconsciously or unconsciously. Sattva allows an individual to remain balanced and avoid swinging between extremes. This does not mean that a sattva-oriented individual will never engage in extremes for temporary periods of time or for specific reasons. However, a sattvic oriented individual will intentionally return to balance when able and will not dwell in extremes unnecessarily.

Rajas is the capacity that the mind utilizes to mobilize, to initialize movement from a resting state, and to maintain and increase activity. Overemphasis of rajas by an individual creates repetitive action without a conscience. An individual may start performing activities simply for the sake of moving or avoiding stillness. Without the presence of tamas, the individual will rarely slow down, ultimately deplete him or herself completely. When sattva is not present, many of an individual's rajasic actions are motivated by subconscious desires.

Tamas is the capacity the mind uses to resist, slow or stop activity. It is not a representation of a resting state. Rather it forcefully works against movement. Overemphasis of tamas by an individual creates stagnancy, suffocating the initiation of mobilization. In the event that an action initiates, the excess tamasic force will resist its movement constantly, creating a drag. Without the presence of rajas, the individual will become dull, stagnant, numb, and ultimately fall into deep depression. When sattva is not present, many of an individual's tamasic tendencies are held in place by unconscious desires.

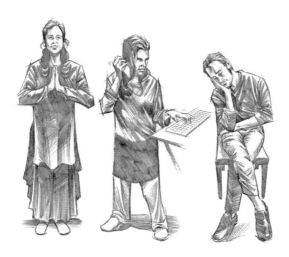

Image 62 - From the Left – Sattva, Rajas and Tamas

Neither rajas nor tamas are inherently detrimental. They are both necessary for creation. When governed by sattva they act harmoniously.

The sleep cycle serves as an example. Tamas is necessary for an individual to gradually reduce nervous system activity from the day into night, withdraw the mind from the sense organs and fall asleep. Rajas is necessary to do the opposite upon waking. A sattva-oriented individual will appropriately apply tamas and rajas to regulate her or his own sleep cycle.

The gunas greatly influence the health of the body. Their graceful or reckless application not only generates immediate effects on the function of the body, but also shapes an individual's entire lifestyle over time.

READING THE SIXTH LAYER OF THE PULSE

The sixth layer of the pulse is read in the same manner as the prakruti layer pulse with three points of potential contact on each fingertip. This layer represents the inherent stability of an individual's mental activity. There is no mental prakruti as there is a bodily prakruti.

The mind can change its basic behaviors and tendencies throughout life. However, it is an extension of the body's prakruti and is heavily influenced by it. Individuals certainly have inherent, sometimes seemingly unchangeable leanings towards combinations of sattva, rajas and tamas. The sixth layer represents these leanings.

In general, the closer this layer is to the prakruti in both the location of crests and qualities expressed by these crests, the more inclined an individual is towards sattva. This patterning represents that the constitution and the mind are harmonious and reflective of each other. The prominence of rajas and tamas are experienced in the qualities expressed by the crests. Dull, sluggish, slow, sticky, cold and feeble qualities signify the presence of more tamas. Sharp, light, fast, hot and forceful qualities signify the presence of more rajas.

A pulse reader relies on sattva in practicing as the qualities of sattva are conducive to the art of pulse reading. The calm, clear, neutral, non-reactive perceptions along with an intention to experience the truth that sattva carries, enables the pulse reader to discern the subtleties within an individual's pulse. Too much influence from rajas or tamas and the pulse reader will either misinterpret information through biases or miss information altogether. The continued practice of pulse reading itself enhances the student's capacity to utilize sattva. The student that pursues a sattva-oriented lifestyle will find his or her pulse reading much improved.

EXAMPLE OF A SIXTH LAYER PULSE

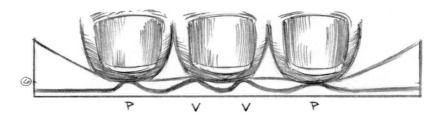

Image 63 - Example of a Sixth Layer Pulse

In the above sixth layer pulse example, suppose that the prakruti pulse matches exactly with the exception of middle finger crests making contact on the kapha and vata locations on the sixth layer. In the prakruti there is a crest making contact at the pitta location in place of the vata location, giving this rogi a true pitta prakruti with kapha as the secondary dosha. In the sixth layer, the crests are, on the whole, expressing pitta qualities with the exception of the middle fingertip crests, which are expressing qualities more vata in nature.

The pulse reader can begin to discern that this individual will have a strong tendency towards sattva as three of the four crests match the prakruti layer. However, there is also a habitual tendency for this individual to apply too much rajas indicated by the vata qualities expressed by the middle fingertip vata crest. The pulse reader can explore the effect of this mental tendency by reading all the layers of the pulse and observing the individual's lifestyle.

COMMON MISTAKE

It is easy to mistake the sixth layer for the seventh layer of the pulse and vice versa. It is a good pulse reading practice to always identify the seventh layer first, then slightly release the pressure of the fingertips to ascend to the sixth layer.

CHAPTER ELEVEN

SATTVA, RAJAS AND TAMAS IN THE MOMENT THE SECOND LAYER OF THE PULSE

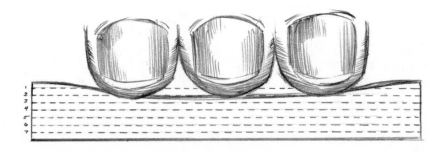

Image 64 - The Second Layer

The second layer of the pulse is read in the same manner as the sixth layer of the pulse. Instead of expressing the deeper, more habitual patterns of the mind, it expresses the mind's utilization of sattva, rajas and tamas in the present moment. It changes with more regularity than the sixth layer and it will likely more closely mirror the vikruti pulse than the prakruti pulse. However, mirroring the vikruti pulse is not a sign of balance. In fact, many imbalances in the vikruti emerge from the sustained, imbalanced utilization of rajas and tamas.

If the second layer pulse has almost no or no similarities to the prakruti pulse, then the pulse reader should become wary of a more severe mental imbalance. It is a signal that the mind is largely disconnected from the functioning of the body. If that same disconnect from the prakruti is found on the sixth layer as well it can be a sign of long-standing mental imbalance.

Differences between the second layer and the sixth layer of the pulse may sometimes seem contradictory. At first it would seem that the tendencies represented by the sixth layer would largely determine the expressions of the second layer. If one guna is prominent in the sixth layer then an individual is likely utilizing it frequently throughout the day, giving rise to its expression on the second layer. This is the case much of the time, but the pulse reader can develop some sophistication in uncovering the roots of the discrepancy between the second and sixth layers. Contained within these differences can be important information regarding the rogi's lifestyle.

For example, on the sixth layer an individual's pulse expresses a heavy tendency towards the utilization of rajas. On the second layer an individual's pulse is expressing a heavy utilization of tamas in complete contradiction to the sixth layer. The pulse reader can begin to suspect that the individual is suffering from 'burnout.' The individual's highly rajasic lifestyle over a long period of time depleted the individual's ojas leaving him or her without the bodily resources to maintain such a high utilization of rajas. The tendencies expressed by the sixth layer remain, though they cannot be acted upon in the moment. However, unless the individual were to change his or her mental tendencies, the moment the individual regains strength, that strength will be spent through the re-engagement of rajas. Tamas will set in again and the cycle will continue.

EXAMPLE OF A SECOND LAYER PULSE

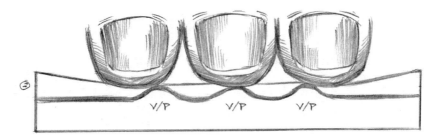

Image 65 - Example of a Second Layer Pulse

In this example, the crests are making contact with the ring fingertip on the vata location, with the middle fingertip on the pitta location,

123

Victor Briere A.D.

and with the index fingertip on the kapha location. All of the crests are primarily expressing vata and pitta qualities. The rogi's prakruti is the same, but with an additional crest on the index fingertip at the vata location expressing the rogi's vata prominent constitution. The rogi's sixth layer pulse differs more from the prakruti than the second layer pulse does and expresses itself quite feebly which suggests more tamasic tendencies. The vikruti, first layer, pulse more closely resembles the sixth layer than it does the second and seventh layers.

In this reading, the pulse reader can identify one of the rogi's core intentions. The pulse reader, intuitively receiving all this information, may begin to understand that this rogi is actively putting forth energy into changing his or her mental tendencies to move away from the utilization of tamas and to match more closely with the prakruti. The second layer pulse is expressing the current efforts of the rogi. Its similarity to the prakruti reveals that the rogi is exercising sattva, command over rajas and tamas. This could take the form of intentionally adopting a more sattvic lifestyle that includes spiritual practices along with wholesome, rhythmic living. If the rogi persists, eventually the sixth layer pulse would express itself more closely to the prakruti, representing a fundamental change in the tendencies of the mind. The vikruti would certainly change as well under the new influence of balanced use of rajas and tamas.

COMMON MISTAKE

Many pulse readers underestimate the physiological impact of mental activities. A rogi may claim they are depressed because they are ill but often it is the other way around. The pulse reader will benefit from understanding a rogi's intentions by reading the second and sixth layers of the pulse. Excessive and underuse of rajas and tamas are primary causes of functional physical imbalances.

124

CHAPTER TWELVE

THE ESSENCES OF THE DOSHAS - PRANA, TEJAS AND OJAS THE FOURTH LAYER OF THE PULSE

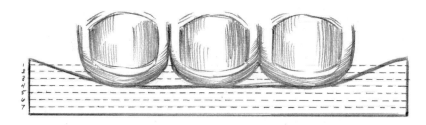

Image 66 - The Fourth Layer

The fourth layer of the pulse is read in the same manner as the seventh layer of the pulse with one exception. Kapha translates to ojas, pitta to tejas, and vata to prana. The fourth layer expresses the presence of the essences of each of the doshas. It is a measure of how well the body refines the physiological doshas of vata, pitta, and kapha and integrates them with the mental gunas of sattva, rajas and tamas. Only an individual who has cultivated sattva appropriately will generate a balance between prana, tejas and ojas.

Prana is the energy that animates an individual's existence. It is the flow of life through, within, and beyond the being. Tejas, at its core, is an individual's ability to broaden or focus his or her attention as desired. The individual can project her or his presence to an entire room, or intensely focus on a particular thought or action. Ojas is a measure of one's physical endurance and resilience. It is the flexible stability that tejas can rely on.

The three can be likened to an oil lantern. Kapha is the fuel contained in the lantern. Ojas is the purity or efficiency of the fuel. Pitta is the flame consuming the oil. Tejas is the light the flame emits broadened or narrowed by the shutters. Vata is the air present within and around the lantern. Prana is the oxygen content in the air, surrounding it wholly and necessary for its existence.

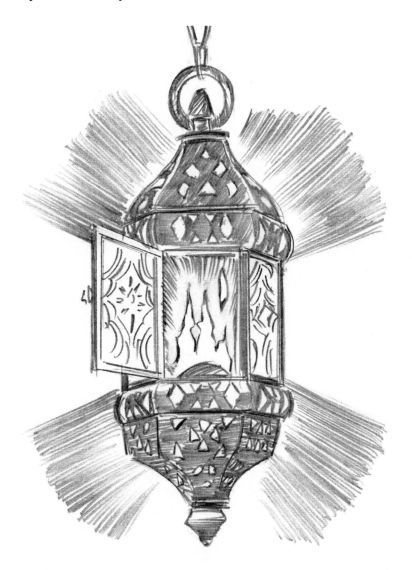

Image 67 - Lantern Representing Prana, Tejas, and Ojas

Inside a person these relationships are the same, but more complex.

The quality of the fuel is comprised of many different bodily components and relies on many different functions. The light emitted from the flame is a complex series of functions that generates intelligence, awareness, intention and attention. The oxygen in the air is all the different sources of energy that exist within and without the body at any given moment.

Prana, tejas and ojas are less fickle than the mental gunas, though their balance is changeable throughout life unlike the prakruti. Since they are refined essences, it takes some time for the body to develop them. In the case of prana, it is readily available everywhere. It does not need to be created by the body. However, the bodily channels must open and flow correctly to harness its limitless energy. In the case of tejas, which is also limitless, the body must refine all of its metabolic processes in order to fully express tejas' presence. In the case of ojas, the body produces it by refining ahara for over one month. The overall quality of ojas is therefore dependent on the quality of each dhatu.

Individuals typically go through periods of life in which one of the three is more prominent. If the individual is focused on healing and rejuvenating the body and just completed panchakarma therapy, ojas will likely be most prominently expressed in the fourth layer. If the individual is focused on being a leader in her or his career for a period of time, tejas will likely be most prominently expressed. If the individual is engaging in a serious yoga and pranayama practice for a period of time, prana will likely be most prominently expressed.

The "prana" as a subdosha of vata is distinct from the "prana" observed on the fourth layer of the pulse. In the context of the subdosha, it mainly refers to the movement and behavior of vata. In the context of tejas and ojas it refers to lifeforce, or, the quality of aliveness. In this sense ayurvedic sages identify thirteen storehouses of prana.

1. The Temples
2. Heart
3. Umbilicus

4. Urinary Bladder
5. Throat
6. Blood Tissue
7. Shukra Dhatu
8. Ojas
9. Anus
10. All Agni
11. Sattva
12. Rajas
13. Tamas

When perfectly balanced, the fourth layer of the pulse will have even crests on all three fingertips. It will express balanced kapha qualities under the ring fingertip, balanced pitta qualities under the middle fingertip and balanced vata qualities under the index fingertip. It need not match the prakruti pulse. This indicates that the individual is living in complete harmony with her or his prakruti. This is a truly rare occasion and seldom achieved. Any other pattern of crests and qualities indicates to the pulse reader from which essence the individual is primarily drawing from.

COMMON PATTERNS IN THE FOURTH LAYER

There are some common patterns the pulse reader will experience as she or he practices. High prana without adequate ojas signals mental instability, gauntness, insomnia and manic, though sometimes highly creative, behavior. If prana is high and tejas is also inadequate, then the individual may feel highly creative but blocked in the expression of it. The individual may also have great creative potential and an abundance of energy but will be unable to focus for any significant length of time such as in attention deficit disorders.

High tejas without sufficient prana creates blind faith, fervor or leadership without a conscience. An individual can possess great leadership qualities but lacks the energy or enthusiasm to carry them out. Tejas is an outward expression and utilizes the body's resources as fuel. High tejas without sufficient ojas depletes the physical body's resources leading to burnout. Ojas is the primary resource that the immune system draws upon. As such, high tejas without ojas can create immune deficiency or autoimmune disorders.

High ojas without sufficient prana creates a desire to simply exist with no other purpose or creative spark. Mundane routine sets in with no evolution or growth. The body can become stagnant over a very long period of time due to habituated self-imposed isolation and a desire to 'hibernate.' High ojas without sufficient tejas creates a similar effect to a high prana with low tejas pattern. The individual is creative but lacks the focus to execute or manifest that creativity. However, in this case, with an abundance of ojas this pattern can maintain itself for many years, even a lifetime.

EXAMPLE OF A FOURTH LAYER PULSE

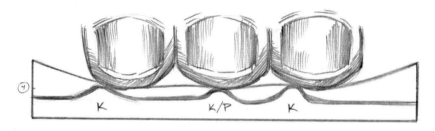

Image 68 - Example of a Fourth Layer Pulse

In this example the crests are making contact on the ring fingertip on the kapha location, the middle fingertip on the pitta location and the index fingertip on the kapha location. The qualities expressed by the crests are primarily those of kapha and pitta. This could be the pulse pattern of an individual going through some type of rejuvenation therapy. The pulse reader may find this outcome if the mental status of the rogi is geared towards sattva at the time of the reading. However, this pulse pattern could also represent a lack of prana flowing through the body, especially if none of the crests express vata qualities, particularly those on the index finger. If the pulse reader ascertains a high level of tamas utilization coupled with excess kapha qualities in the other layers of the pulse, he or she should become wary of prana depletion.

COMMON MISTAKE

Many pulse readers consider the absence of a crest related to one of the essences to be a sign of depletion of that essence. This could certainly be true. However, the absence of a crest alone is not enough to signify genuine depletion. The pulse reader should pay attention to other indications of depletion associated with that essence on other layers of the pulse before arriving at such a conclusion.

CHAPTER THIRTEEN

READING AND ASSESSING THE NAVEL PULSE AND OTHER USEFUL PULSE READING SITES

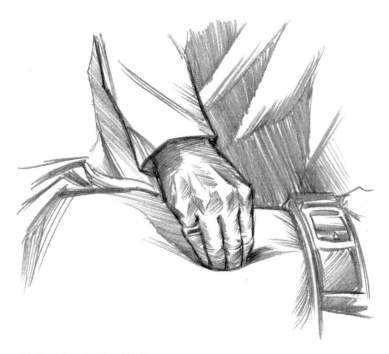

Image 69 - Reading the Navel Pulse

The radial artery is the main site of pulse reading for the practitioner. However, there are other important locations from which to ascertain knowledge. The navel is one of them. It is the original source of nourishment for the body while in the mother's womb. The navel pulse is felt just underneath or around the umbilicus with all five fingers. To read a rogi's navel pulse, the rogi should lay on his or her back as in savasana, corpse pose. The rogi should be directed to take a few deep abdominal breaths and then fully exhale and hold the exhale while the pulse reader pushes downward with all five fingertips on the center of the umbilicus.

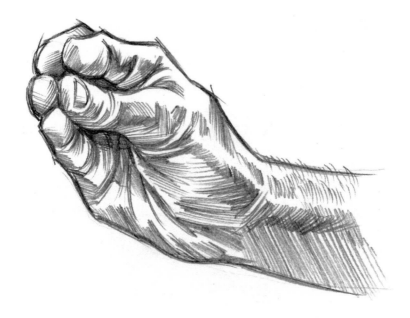

Image 70 - Navel Pulse Fingertip Form

If the navel pulse is expressing balance, the pulse reader will feel a strong, steady, pulsation centered *directly underneath* the point where all five fingers meet at the direct center of the umbilicus. If the navel pulse is expressing imbalance it will be absent, feeble, or extremely forceful. It can also be off-center. Frequently, its resonance can be felt inches away from the umbilicus.

The navel pulse primarily expresses three major capacities. The strength of overall digestion, the ability for an individual to remain emotionally balanced, and willpower. These three capacities are inextricable connected. Emotionality, whether suppressed or overexpressed has a vast and prominent effect on the entire nervous system, and especially the digestion. When a person is threatened, triggered or in fear, the sympathetic nervous system is engaged, and the digestive process slows to a halt. Willpower is the fruit of both emotional balance and digestive strength. Sustained efforts fueled by willpower are protected by physical robustness and emotional resilience. The individual remains unperturbed in the face of distractions and challenges.

If the navel pulse is felt anywhere outside the center of the umbilicus it is signaling some form of emotional distress and some form of digestive disturbance. The two almost always go together. Emotionally, it could indicate fear, anger, anxiety, depression, disingenuous positivity, etc. In the digestive system it could indicate, diarrhea, constipation, alternation between diarrhea and constipation, flatulence, excessive belching, malabsorption of nourishment, etc.

These digestive issues herald a host of other issues. Once the digestive system becomes impaired, the collapse of wellbeing is imminent.

COMMON MISTAKE

The pulse reader may find it challenging to insert the five fingers directly on the center of the umbilicus. It is common that the pulse reader's hand becomes skewed in the process, making a centered pulse appear proximal or vice versa. To avoid this, the pulse reader may place the fingertips just above the umbilicus to ensure that they are perpendicular prior to inserting them into the navel.

OTHER USEFUL PULSE READING SITES

The pulse reader may choose to check a local pulse if he or she identifies a particular area of imbalance in the body. While it would not typically be appropriate to read the layers of each local pulse, assessing the local pulse for general doshic qualities can provide a good deal of information regarding localized doshic activity.

PULSE READING SITES ACROSS THE BODY

LOCATION	DESCRIPTION
TEMPORAL	CENTER OF THE TEMPLES
ORBITAL	IN BETWEEN THE TWO EYEBROWS OR ON EITHER SIDE OF THE NOSE JUST BELOW THE EYEBROWS
CAROTID	ON THE NECK BELOW THE ANGLE OF THE JAW LINE ON EITHER SIDE OF THE JUGULAR
AXILLARY	CENTER OF THE ARMPIT SLIGHTLY TOWARDS THE FRONT OF THE BODY
BRACHIAL	INSIDE OF THE ELBOW ON THE ULNAR SIDE OVER THE BICEP TENDON
FEMORAL	NEXT TO THE PUBIC BONE IN THE INGUINAL AREA ON THE INSIDE OF THE THIGH
POSTERIOR TIBIAL	BETWEEN THE INSIDE ANKLE BONE AND THE ACHILLES TENDON

CHAPTER FOURTEEN

READING A PREGNANCY IN THE PULSE

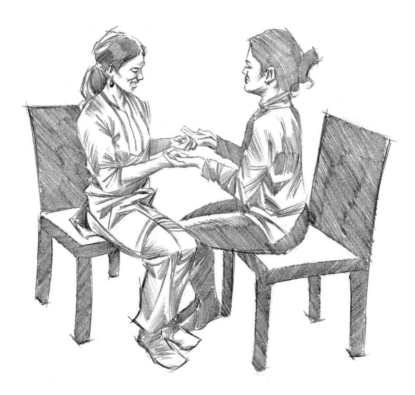

Image 71 - Reading a Pregnancy in the Pulse

As the pulse reader delves through the layers of a female rogi's pulse he or she may come across a highly active shukra/arthava dhatu on the fifth layer pulse expressing primarily kapha and then pitta qualities. The vikruti may also express more kapha and pitta qualities than present in the prakruti. The fourth layer of the pulse may express an increased generation of ojas. The third layer of pulse may express more activity from prana vata, vyana vata, samana vata, pachaka pitta, avalambaka kapha, and tarpaka kapha. This can prompt the pulse reader to inquire about the menstrual cycle. The rogi may be experiencing menses, ovulation, or pregnancy.

If after reading the radial artery pulse, the pulse reader suspects that the individual may be pregnant, the pulse reader may read the interior of both pinkies simultaneously, below the first knuckle, with the pads of his or her thumbs.

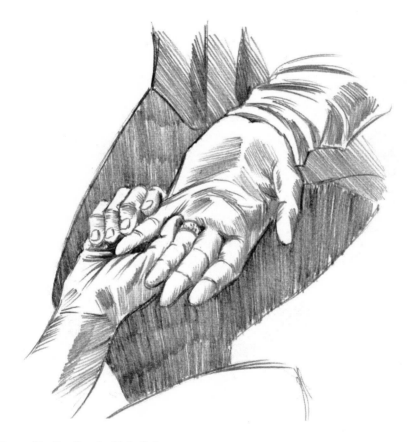

Image 72 - Reading the Pinky Pulses

This pulse will be more robust than usual *relative* to the pregnant individual's pulse when not pregnant. It will likely express more kapha and pitta qualities. This increased amplitude, force and breadth occurs within weeks of conception as the woman's body begins to change its patterns to provide for the new life.

After four to five months the pulse reader may find that one of the pinky pulses is more robust than the other. This is a loose indication of the sex of the child. More often than not, a more robust pulse on the left pinky heralds a girl and the right, a boy. Often the distinction between pinky pulses becomes more prominent in the third trimester.

COMMON MISTAKE

The most common mistake when reading a female's pulse is to completely overlook the possibility that she may be pregnant. Without this possibility in mind, the pulse reader may interpret the pulse as imbalanced and proceed as such. Depending on the course of healing, this can be dangerous for both the mother and the fetus.

CHAPTER FIFTEEN

COMMUNICATING FINDINGS TO THE ROGI

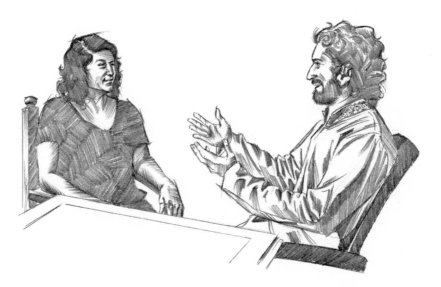

Image 73 - Open Communication

The pulse reader is a translator on behalf of the body. Most of the time, a rogi approaches the pulse reader because the body is expressing that something is out of balance via symptoms. The rogi, in an attempt to do away with the discomfort, seeks out aid.

It is not simply the pulse reader's task to identify and confirm symptoms. It is the pulse reader's task to truly listen to the body's cry for help and unveil the origin of the imbalance.

The pulse reader takes what was unveiled from listening to the expression of the pulse and translates that to the rogi so that the rogi may understand what his or her own body is communicating beyond the suffering of symptoms. Often, the root issue on its own does not generate symptoms. For example, high blood sugar levels in and of themselves do not cause a rogi discomfort. The damage caused to the tissues by high blood sugar in time is what the rogi experiences, and only when that damage becomes severe enough. Yet the danger to the body is present long before the symptoms manifest.

A rogi in his or her sympathetic nervous system will have more difficulty understanding and accepting the pulse reader's assessment as truth. In the modern era, with the existence of varieties of ultrasounds, X-rays, CAT scans, MRI's, blood panels etc., there is often a measure of skepticism regarding pulse reading as an accurate method of assessing the body. The pulse reader should not be deterred by this skepticism but should certainly be aware that he or she is often up against it and consider this in the communication of her or his findings. It is often the case that a pulse reader can identify imbalances that other types of tests cannot. It is also important for the pulse reader to remember that many of the modern tests need to be interpreted by a professional, and the accuracy of those interpretations is dependent on many of the same skills the pulse reader utilizes, namely, discernment, attention, intuitive understanding, and listening. Accuracy is one component of communication but there are other aspects of communication that are just as vital.

The manner in which the pulse reader communicates the findings to a rogi influences the physiology of the rogi, and thus the pulses.

It is usually more digestible for the rogi, and more informative for the pulse reader, to discuss the findings as a dialogue as opposed to a lecture. Presenting the findings in one uninterrupted speech does not allow a rogi to comment or contribute more information to the findings.

NEUTRALITY

The pulse reader must deliver findings neutrally. Neutrality does not mean disconnected, flat or monotone. This means that the pulse reader should not become enmeshed with his or her personal emotions and biases surrounding the findings. It is why it is more difficult to read the pulses of a loved one. There are some healing traditions that heavily caution against taking on the role of the healer for someone in the immediate family. Becoming truly neutral is an enormous feat in and of itself. To add a familial component to this makes an already difficult task nearly impossible.

If the pulse reader does react to a finding for one reason or another, then the pulse reader should recognize this and reconsider his or her findings. The pulse reader can pause, take a breath, and read the pulses again. The danger is not in having biases or reactions, these are inevitable. The danger is in not realizing they are present and going one step further, representing them as truth.

CONFIDENCE

The findings can be communicated with perfect accuracy and with beautiful language, but if they are not delivered with confidence then they will likely make little impact. In the art of pulse reading, confidence emerges from a mixture of discipline, self-esteem, experience, knowledge, humility and compassion. False confidence is typically detectible by a carefully listening rogi, especially a skeptical one. The pulse reader must genuinely believe in her or his experience of the findings. This inner solidity forms the support for the ensuing dialogue.

Even uncertainty regarding findings can be delivered with confidence. There are bound to be communications within the pulse that the pulse reader does not understand at the time of the reading. This is not a reason to engage in self-doubt. So long as the pulse reader has other findings to offer, he or she can simply communicate, with confidence, that there are certain aspects of the reading that were unclear and require more exploration.

COMPASSION

The pulse reader should practice delivering findings with compassion. This serves many purposes. Highest among these is the essential motivation for practicing the art of pulse reading to begin with, which is to aid in a rogi's healing. Compassion also carries a special quality that can penetrate a rogi's defense mechanisms. If a rogi senses compassion, it helps him or her feel safe, at least in the long run, moving the rogi into her or his parasympathetic nervous system so that the body can rejuvenate. The compassionate intentions of the pulse reader can open the door to a long-term, trusting relationship which is essential in the effectiveness of all healing modalities.

Much of the time, rogis are reacting and responding less to what the pulse reader is saying, and more to the perceived quality of the pulse reader's character. In so much as the pulse reader is reading the rogi, the rogi is reading the pulse reader.

If the rogi senses that the pulse reader is genuinely there to help _and_ that the pulse reader is confident, the rogi will be much more willing to accept the findings as accurate, and more importantly, adopt the suggestions that will help him or her heal.

DISCERNMENT

There are findings that are relevant to the rogi's healing and there are findings that, while reliable, are not relevant. It is up to the pulse reader discern which findings to deliver and in what manner to deliver them. It is not useful, and potentially harmful, to tell an already anxious rogi all of the possible imbalances present and all of the possible chronic ailments that can develop in the future. Alternately, if a rogi is overly confident regarding his or her resilience, it can be important to deliver more information regarding the state of imbalance and its severity.

The rogi may need to be addressed very directly. The rogi may need to be addressed very gently. There is a myriad of ways to go about conveying the same information. Compassion is the best guide for discernment, as the discernment must be based on the intention to help the rogi heal and not on an ulterior motive.

CLARITY

The pulse reader needs to communicate to the rogi in a manner that the rogi can understand. Using too much Sanskrit terminology or attempting to explain complex ayurvedic concepts can leave most rogis feeling blank, confused and unsupported. Communicating the finding that, "Due to excess rajas in your dinacharya, samana vata is aggravated, leading to aggravated apana vata, which has created a generalized vata imbalance localizing in the majja dhatu ultimately leading to a degradation of tarpaka kapha resulting in chronic loss of muscle control," is generally not useful to a rogi. This can be rephrased and customized in such a way that the rogi genuinely understands what is unfolding inside her or his body.

VALIDATION

As a holistic science, Ayurveda encourages the utilization of all of the pulse reader's senses in order to validate the findings of the pulse reading. Pulse diagnosis should never be used in isolation from other diagnostic techniques.

Findings should be supported and cross-referenced primarily through darshana, sparshana, and prashna.

Darshana refers to the use of sight in order to assess the rogi's prakruti, vikruti, gait, skin condition, hair condition, how they are dressed, facial expressions, body language, etc. Sparshana refers to the use of touch in order to assess the rogi's status. It includes the technique of palpation to feel the aspects of the body that cannot be seen, such as the internal organs. It also includes feeling the texture and temperature of the skin.

Prashna is the art of asking the rogi direct and indirect questions in order to uncover missing or hidden information, to confirm or deny what has already been observed, or to gather more details regarding a particular point of interest. It is one of the most important diagnostic tools at the pulse reader's disposal and inseparable from the practice of pulse reading.

When what is experienced via darshana, sparshana and prashna validates the findings of the pulse reading it is a strong indicator of confirmation. However, if what is experienced does not reflect the findings of the pulse reading, it does not mean one or the other is necessarily innacurate. Rather, it represents an important area that requires deeper investigation, *usually through prashna*. Often times, these seemingly dissenting observations are individual pieces of an incomplete puzzle pointing the way to the true nature of an imbalance.

PAY CLOSE ATTENTION TO BODY LANGUAGE

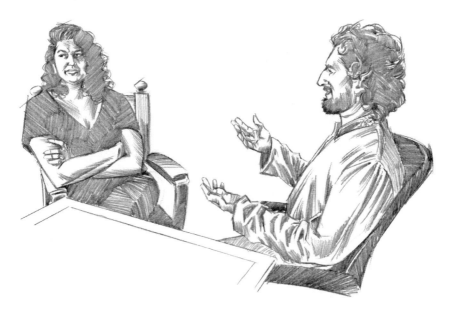

Image 74 - Closed Communication

The rogi may be nodding her or his head in agreement and saying "yes" to all of the pulse reader's suggestions, but the crossed legs, crossed arms, lack of eye contact and general attitude of rejection are communicating otherwise. Reading body language is an art unto itself. The pulse reader must be attentive to certain overt cues while communicating to track the recipient's experience. The pulse reader may have been informed about a rogi's fearful or defensive disposition by the pulses themselves and the body language may reconfirm this.

The pulse reader may be delivering difficult information that triggers the rogi's defenses. The rogi may not trust the pulse reader yet. The rogi may have just had a conflict with his or her spouse about paying for the consultation. Whatever the reason, if the rogi is defensive then communication and adoption of healthy suggestions will be stunted dramatically.

COMMUNICATING THROUGH THE FEELING OF THREAT

If the rogi is communicating vocally or through body language that he or she is not receptive, then it does not behoove either the rogi or the pulse reader for the pulse reader to continue explaining the findings. In truth, doing so can actually damage the relationship as the rogi may not feel acknowledged or listened to. This undermines a trusting relationship.

Countless techniques have been explored and developed to communicate through threat over the centuries. There is no single universal technique that works with everyone. The "use" of a technique as a means to convey safety can even be construed as a threat in certain situations. The pulse reader will need to use discernment within each situation as it presents itself. If appropriate, the pulse reader can inquire as to what is creating a sense of dis-ease in the rogi. It is rare that the rogi will directly reveal the exact reason for dis-ease, either because the rogi doesn't know him or herself, or because he or she is unwilling to share. However, the pulse reader's willingness to attempt to understand can go a long way and potentially bear the fruits of trust in the future.

COMMON MISTAKE

Many pulse readers genuinely listen to the pulse and reliably ascertain the true nature of the prakruti and imbalances. Believing their job is complete, they do not put forth their best effort in communicating those findings, which leaves the rogi feeling empty or confused. The student of the pulse should consider the communication of the findings as part of the pulse reading itself, never breaking focus until the entire session is concluded.

CHAPTER SIXTEEN

PUTTING IT ALL TOGETHER – READING ALL SEVEN LAYERS

With the knowledge of how to read the seven layers of the pulse and the organ pulses, the pulse reader can form a holistic understanding of the relevant, pertinent workings of an individual's body. There are as many ways to synthesize the information gained from the pulses as there are pulse readers.

AN ORDER OF READING THE LAYERS

There is not one correct protocol for the order of reading the layers of the pulse. The only steadfast "rule" is to read the prakruti layer first as it creates a context for all of the other information communicated by the pulse. It is generally easier to ascend from the deeper layers than to begin at a shallower layer and delve downwards. Below are a few orderings that the student of the pulse can practice with. The student will likely have an affinity for one and readily adopt as his or her standard.

DELVE THEN SURFACE

The pulse reader begins by reading the prakruti layer. From there she or he surfaces all the way to the vikruti layer. From that point, delves to the prakruti layer again only as a reference to find the sixth layer. Once the sixth layer is read, surfaces momentarily to the first layer and from which finds the second layer. Back down to the prakruti layer momentarily, then ascends to the fifth layer. From the fifth layer it is relatively simple to reach the third layer, and finally the fourth layer. After reading all of the layers, the pulse reader begins to read the organ pulses, beginning with the first layer and delving to the seventh layer, repeating this with each finger on one hand, and then switching to the other.

An advantage to this method is that the pulse reader can compare the vikruti layer with the prakruti layer immediately. The same goes for the sixth and second layers.

DELVE THEN ASCEND

The pulse reader begins by reading the prakruti layer. From there he or she ascends one layer at a time in succession. Once all the layers have been observed, the pulse reader reads the organ pulses.

An advantage to this method is that the pulse reader can easily experience which crests remain consistent through all the layers while engrossed in the reading, and not afterwards by reviewing findings. This can yield a sense of understanding of a common thread through all the layers and provide special insight into the samprapti of an imbalance.

ORGANS FIRST

The pulse reader begins by reading the organ pulses prior to engaging in one of the prior two methods. Some pulse readers prefer this because they find it useful to understand the body in terms of the vital organs first, and then the more functional aspects.

FUNCTION FOCUSED

The pulse reader begins by reading the organ pulses. The pulse reader then delves down to read the prakruti layer, ascends to the vikruti layer for reference, and then goes immediately to the third layer and reads the subdoshic activity. The pulse reader then carries on reading the other layers of the pulse through the lens of subdoshic and organ activity.

An advantage to this method is the simplicity and clarity it provides in assessing the more functional aspects of the body. It can be performed as an adjunct pulse reading after a more complete pulse reading has been carried out. In this way, the pulse reader can focus on a particular set of functions inside the body.

FIRST LAYER ONLY

This is a traditional form of pulse reading that is written about in select ayurvedic texts. Those texts do not describe engaging in the observation of multiple layers. Rather, the complete focus is on the qualities, gait, rate, rhythm and force found in the first layer. If there is an overall feeling of balance in the pulse, then it can be understood that the rogi is in alignment with her or his prakruti.

An advantage to this method is its efficiency. Seasoned pulse readers can receive an abundance of information from the first layer alone. Since the first layer expresses the rogi's holistic, current bodily state, some consider it the most relevant layer to assessing imbalance.

SAMPRAPTI

Both of the below cases serve to illuminate how a pulse reader can uncover the *samprapti* of an imbalance. The samprapti is the pathology of a disease. The pulse reader can follow the root cause of an imbalance from its origins to the presenting symptoms. The basic steps of a samprapti are as follows:

1. Accumulation – The doshas begin to accumulate in their respective seats.
2. Provocation – The doshas become agitated within their seats and begin to function abnormally. This begins to impair the balanced generation of dhatus.
3. Spread – The doshas become uncontained in their seats and begin to spread throughout the body in an unnatural manner.
4. Localization – The aggravated and excess doshas are deposited into weakened dhatus and organs, further weakening and damaging the dhatus and organs.
5. Manifestation – The weakened and damaged dhatus and organs begin to change their form, underlying structure, and function.

6. Differentiation – The improper functioning and altered structure of the dhatus and organs creates weaknesses and damage in other areas of the body. The circulating, aggravated doshas localize there as well, creating a new manifestation stage, and potentially another differentiation. At this stage, the cessation of the root cause may not necessarily reverse the samprapti.

EXAMPLE OF A COMPLETE PULSE READING "MANDY"

Sex: Female
Age: 27
Height: 5'5"
Weight: 140lbs
Occupation: Real Estate Agent
Relationship Status: Single
Children: None
Appointment Time: 8:00am

Mandy's primary complaints are excess weight, occasional acid reflux and fatigue on a daily basis, especially after eating. Upon walking in the room, the pulse reader suspects that she has a kapha and pitta prominent prakruti based on her bone structure and facial features. After a brief introduction and conversation regarding her reasons for coming, the pulse reader requests Mandy's left wrist. She reaches out but with a hesitance. Noticing this, the pulse reader asks if she has ever had her pulses read. She shyly responds that she has, only in a doctor's office from a nurse. While guiding her arm to be supported by the desk, the pulse reader explains that ayurvedic pulse reading is a little different, that it will take a few minutes, and that she can just relax and breathe. Mandy smiles, feeling acknowledged, and relaxes the tension in her arm.

MANDY'S PULSES

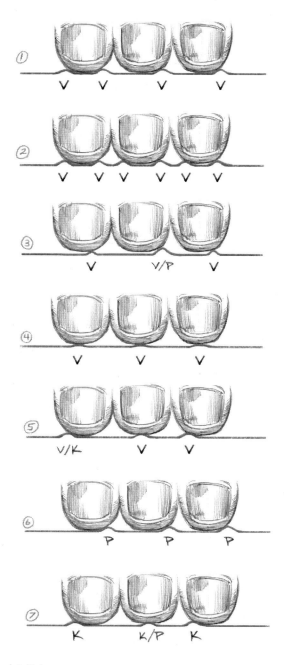

Image 75 - Mandy's Pulses

Gently placing the fingertips on her left wrist, the pulse reader's immediate impression is that vata is aggravated based on the narrow string-like expression of the overall pulse especially in the context of the suspected prakruti. Before assessing the first layer further, the pulse reader delves to the seventh layer.

The seventh layer confirms the suspected prakruti. Two of the crests contact the kapha location of the fingertips and one on the pitta location on the middle fingertip. Kapha and pitta are in their natural locations. The qualities expressed in the crests are soft and rounded. The rate is moderate, about 65 beats per minute. The gait feels like water rolling across the crest at the point of contact suggesting a kapha nature. The force is ample suggesting a pitta nature. The volume is full, again suggesting a kapha nature. The texture and quality of the artery itself is quite elastic and broad suggesting a kapha nature. The surface temperature of the skin is cool, but also very slightly clammy. The pulse reader takes note of this.

The rhythm is very steady. At this point the pulse reader makes a point to check for a respiratory sinus arrhythmia and asks Mandy to take a deep breath, hold it briefly and then exhale fully. There is absolutely no change in her pulse rate. The pulse reader asks her to repeat the breath. Again, absolutely no change in pulse rate. In the pulse reader's self-talk the connection is made between the prakruti, the complete absence of a respiratory sinus arrhythmia and the initial impression of the pulse expressing such a dramatic vata quality in the context of a kapha-pitta prominent prakruti.

The pulse reader surfaces to the first layer to listen to the vikruti expression more thoroughly. The ring fingertip is contacted by two crests, one in the kapha location and one in the vata location. The kapha crest matches the prakruti in location but is expressing vata qualities. The vata crest is weaker and feels like a pinprick. The middle fingertip is contacted by a crest in the vata location and is expressing itself through a feeble pinprick as well. The index fingertip is contacted by a crest in the vata location and is expressing another pinprick, though with more strength than the middle finger. The only crest that aligns with the prakruti is the kapha crest on the ring finger and even that crest does not match in quality of expression. With the confidence that the overall vikruti is expressing a systemic, prominent, vata imbalance, the pulse reader delves to the seventh layer momentarily for reference, and then ascends to the sixth layer of the pulse.

The sixth layer of the pulse shares the force of the seventh layer but the quality of rolling across the crests on the fingertips is replaced by a much sharper decline, suggesting a pitta quality. The crests on each of the fingertips make contact in the vata location. None of the crests align with the prakruti suggesting that the tendency of her mind is not to utilize sattva but to primarily utilize rajas. Taking note of this the pulse reader ascends to the first layer for reference and then delves into the second layer.

The second layer of the pulse shares the same vata qualities of expression as the first layer. The most striking feature of this layer is the presence of two crests making contact on each fingertip. One on the kapha location and one on the vata location. This suggests that Mandy is presently experiencing swings between rajas and tamas regularly. Since her mind inherently leans towards the utilization of rajas, the pulse reader makes note of the importance of the presence of tamasic tendencies in the progression of the systemic vata imbalance. From here, the pulse reader delves to the third layer.

In the third layer the pulse reader experiences a crest making contact on the portion of the fingertip correlating to avalambaka kapha. It is expressing vata qualities as narrow and slightly feeble. The middle finger crest is making contact on the portion of the fingertip correlating to pachaka pitta. It is expressing the same vata qualities but is slightly more robust. The index finger crest is making contact on the portion of the fingertip correlating to udana vata. Again, expressing the vata qualities of narrowness and feebleness. Without jumping to conclusions, the pulse reader notes the relationship between active udana vata, pachaka pitta and avalambaka kapha, especially in the context of acid reflux. The pulse reader delves past the fourth layer and into the fifth layer.

151

The fifth layer of the pulse feels rounded as in the prakruti but also less robust. In comparison to the breadth and fullness of the prakruti, it feels slightly empty, communicating the presence of a higher proportion of the akash element in the dhatus than the prakruti would naturally generate. The crest on the ring finger is making contact at the location correlating to the rasa dhatu. It is expressing the roundedness of kapha but is feeble and hollow feeling as if wind were rolling across the crest and not water. The crest on the middle finger is making contact at one of the locations correlating to shukra dhatu. It is barely perceptible. The pulse reader is unsure if it is a crest at all. The crest on the index finger is making contact at the location corresponding to asthi dhatu and is less hollow feeling, but narrow and ephemeral. The pulse reader takes note of the continued confirmation of a systemic vata imbalance and becomes wary of a fairly severe nutritional deficiency given the involvement of the rasa dhatu, the weakness of the shukra dhatu and the vata aggravation effecting even the asthi dhatu, which is highly resilient to degradation caused by vata. The pulse reader also remembers that Mandy is only 27 years old and of a kapha-pitta prominent constitution. For there to be this level of depletion in her body means that the issues are quite chronic and ongoing. From here, the pulse reader ascends to the fourth layer.

In the fourth layer of the pulse, the three crests are making contact with the fingertips with such little force that they are barely perceptible. The pulse can be felt, but it is as if the crests can't be pinned down to a specific location and are dispersed across the entire fingertip. With difficulty, the pulse reader makes out that the ring finger crest is making contact at the kapha location of the fingertip. The middle finger crest also makes contact at the kapha location of the fingertip. The index finger crest makes contact at pitta location of the fingertip. The ring finger crest is in alignment with the prakruti in location but expressing such little force that it indicates a deficiency in the body's creation of ojas. The middle finger crest is not in alignment with the prakruti and also communicates a meek attempt to generate ojas. The index finger crest, also not in alignment with the prakruti, is expressing a deficiency in the utilization of tejas. The pulse reader takes note of the confirmation this communicates regarding depletion. The pulse reader also takes note of how shyly and tensely Mandy presented herself confirming a deficiency in the utilization of tejas. With all the layers read, the pulse reader moves on to reading the organ pulses.

MANDY'S ORGAN PULSES

LEFT RADIAL ARTERY			RIGHT RADIAL ARTERY		
ORGAN	CREST LOCATION	QUALITY	ORGAN	CREST LOCATION	QUALITY
SMALL INTESTINE	VATA	VATA	COLON	PITTA	VATA/KAPHA
HEART	VATA	PITTA	LUNGS	KAPHA	PITTA/KAPHA
STOMACH	NONE	VATA	GALLBLADDER	NONE	NONE
SPLEEN & PANCREAS	PITTA	PITTA/KAPHA	LIVER	KAPHA/PITTA	KAPHA/PITTA
BLADDER	KAPHA	VATA	PERICARDIUM	VATA	VATA
KIDNEYS	KAPHA/VATA	KAPHA/VATA	CIRCULATION	PITTA	PITTA

The pulse reader removes the middle and ring fingers from the rogi's wrist and moves the index finger to the first layer to read the pulse correlating to the small intestine. The crest makes contact with the fingertip in the vata location. It feels ephemeral, lightly touching the fingertip and then quickly disappearing. The pulse reader then delves down to the seventh layer to read the pulse associated with the heart. The crest is making contact in the vata location but feel stronger and more robust than the small intestine pulse. It is expressing more pitta qualities. The pulse reader takes note that the small intestine pulse is the weaker of the two, but that both are expressing the same systemic vata imbalance.

The pulse reader then removes the index finger from the wrist and moves the middle finger to the first layer corresponding with the stomach. The pulse is extremely weak with no clearly discernable crest. Delving down to the seventh layer the pulse reader hones in on the pulse corresponding to the spleen and pancreas. The crest is making contact on the pitta location of the fingertip and is feels full, forceful and prominent. The spleen and pancreas seem to be functioning in a healthy manner.

Removing the middle finger, the pulse reader then switches to the ring finger and places it on the first layer of the pulse corresponding to the bladder. Unlike in the vikruti pulse the crest is making contact only on the kapha location of the fingertip. It is expressing a narrow, thready quality representing vata once again. Delving to the seventh layer corresponding with the kidneys, the pulse reader finds the crest making contact again in the kapha location but also in the vata location of the fingertip. The qualities expressed by the crest at the kapha location are heavy and the pulse feels like it lingers for a moment before moving forward. The qualities expressed by the crest at the vata location are less prominent and feel like a forceful pinprick.

Before moving to the rogi's right wrist, the pulse reader takes note of the fact that the stomach, small intestine, bladder and kidneys seems to be the most impaired. The presence of such a distinct vata aggravation in the stomach and small intestine suggest significant agni vitiation. This would produce ama immediately after eating, which also ties into the findings regarding the rasa dhatu. Bladder function is strained and the bladder itself is likely suffering from the accumulation of unreleased ama. The kapha vitiation apparent in the kidneys supports this because the kidneys play a large role in filtering ama out of the body. The vata vitiation apparent in the kidneys expresses their struggle to function under the pronounced influence of vata throughout the body.

The pulse reader request Mandy's right wrist which she offers willingly. Before complete disengaging from the left wrist, the pulse reader takes the opportunity to read both pulses simultaneously. They feel relatively balanced from left to right in rate, force and volume. The pulse reader then moves his or her primary pulse reading hand over to Mandy's right wrist.

The pulse reader briefly checks in on the prakruti layer and the vikruti layer to see if they mirror the left pulse. Indeed, they do so the pulse reader feels confident enough to begin checking the organs associated with the right radial artery and skip reading all the layers of the pulse on the right wrist.

The pulse reader removes the middle and ring fingers from Mandy's wrist and places the index finger on the first layer corresponding to the colon. The crest is on the pitta location of the fingertip but certainly feeble, narrow and feels slimy, as though there is a subtle wriggle in it as the crest peaks. Delving to the seventh layer corresponding to the lungs, the pulse reader finds them to be almost surprisingly balanced. The crest is located on the kapha location of the fingertip and feels full, strong and defined.

The index finger comes off the wrist and the middle finger is placed on the first layer corresponding to the gallbladder. There is no pulse at all. The pulse reader is tempted to apply more pressure to see if the pulse appears but decides against it. On no other location of the first layer has the pulse been absent so its absence here is communicating a significant gallbladder issue. Delving to the seventh layer corresponding to the liver, the pulse reader finds a crest at the kapha and pitta locations of the fingertip. The crest on the kapha location feels sticky and sluggish and the crest on the pitta location is extremely forceful, pounding and sharp. The pulse reader takes note that with a severely impaired gallbladder pulse, the liver needs to work harder to perform its functions. The liver pulse is expressing signs of accumulated ama and hyperactive liver function. With the other primary digestive organs straining under the influence of excess vata, the liver is on overdrive.

The pulse reader removes the middle finger and applies the ring finger to the first layer of the pulse corresponding to the pericardium. The crest is found on the vata location of the fingertip. It is expressing vata qualities, feeling feeble and narrow. The pulse reader recalls the vata aggravated activity of avalambaka kapha on the third layer of the pulse of which the pericardium is primarily formed. Delving to the seventh layer corresponding to circulation, the pulse reader finds a crest on the pitta location of the fingertip with moderate strength and no clear indications of agitation.

155

DISCUSSING THE FINDINGS

The pulse reader takes a final moment to synthesize all that was felt, takes a breath, and releases Mandy's wrist. One final connection becomes apparent to the pulse reader. For her height and prakruti she is not overweight. Yet one of Mandy's primary reasons for seeking aid is to lose weight. The pulse reader sits back and pauses before engaging Mandy with the findings. Using *discernment,* the pulse reader decides to ask a few questions prior to unveiling what was found in the pulse reading.

The pulse reader begins by asking a number of questions about Mandy's lifestyle. The time she wakes up, her exercise routine, when she eats, what she eats, when she drinks water, how much alcohol, coffee or other harsh substances she consumes and how regularly, what time she goes to bed, general stress levels, etc.

Strangely enough, Mandy appears to be living quite an impeccable lifestyle. She wakes up at 5am each morning like clockwork to perform a yoga and pranayama practice. She is also training to become a yoga instructor. She has a bowel movement shortly after waking that usually feels complete. She eats fruit or a small bowl of oatmeal for breakfast at 7:30am. She goes to work and makes sure she takes a break from the computer every hour. She has lunch at 12:30pm sharp each day and is able to eat a fresh, hot, organic vegetarian meal because her office has a kitchenette. She eats a light dinner at 6pm and nothing after dinner. At night she reads, performs some light pranayama and then baths before bed. She is in bed, asleep by 10pm. She doesn't drink coffee, and rarely drinks alcohol, less than once per month. She doesn't smoke cigarettes, doesn't use marijuana and doesn't engage in any other drug use. She has no history of unusual familial or ancestral disorders that she is aware of. She is not taking any prescription medications either. She has been living this way since she was eighteen years old and left her home to attend college. The pulses do not reflect a lifestyle of this quality for someone of her age and background.

The pulses don't lie. There is something she is holding back.

The dissonance between the findings and Mandy's lifestyle does not shake the pulse reader's *confidence* in the findings. The pulse reader begins to communicate what he or she has discovered. Realizing that Mandy is hiding something important to her own healing process, the pulse reader *compassionately* understands how hard it must be for Mandy to express what is going on. She is probably feeling a great deal of shame and fear surrounding the potential consequences of her secret becoming public or known within her closest circles.

The pulse reader checks in on him or herself to see if any reactions or biases have been triggered. Feeling *neutral*, the pulse reader *discerns* that Mandy could benefit from a gentle but *clear* description of what her pulses are expressing, prior to questioning Mandy about the incongruence between the pulses and her projection of an impeccable lifestyle.

Even though Mandy revealed that she has some basic knowledge of Ayurveda and yoga, the pulse reader decides to limit the use of ayurvedic terminology as he or she is unsure of the depth of Mandy's knowledge. The pulse reader explains that there is a significant disturbance and weakness in her stomach, small intestine and gallbladder. Her digestion seems to be severely hampered in the upper gastrointestinal tract and because of this her liver is working extremely hard to compensate. Her colon, kidneys and bladder are confirming signs that she is not digesting food properly, leaving ama in her body that isn't being fully released. Overall, the pulses express that all of this is primarily being caused by aggravated vata, resulting in significant depletion throughout her body. The pulse reader pauses to observe Mandy. Mandy seems to be waiting for the pulse reader to keep going.

The pulse reader uses this as an opportunity to insert the most prominent provocative finding of the reading. The pulse reader expresses to Mandy that with her quality of life, all her healthy practices and her health history something seems to be missing. The pulse reader asks Mandy if anything else is going on that she could possibly think of, and then pauses.

Mandy is silent for some time, her gaze cast downward. The pulse reader can tell she is struggling and reminds Mandy that everything said in the session is completely confidential. Mandy explains that she just wants to lose some weight and feel better. The pulse reader *discerns* that it would be best to remain silent and not engage in surface level commentary or to console Mandy. After another moment, Mandy takes a breath and reveals that she has been binging and purging since she was sixteen years old.

The pulse reader and Mandy continue on with the session in the context of this revelation. They are able to have an honest conversation, create deeper threads of trust, and address the underlying issues of her imbalances.

After Mandy leaves, the pulse reader reviews the findings for his or her own benefit. The imbalance of udana vata and pachaka pitta correlates perfectly to the long-standing behavior of vomiting, the acid reflux and even the good health of the lungs. While not healthy for Mandy overall, vomiting can help clean the lungs. The health of her lungs could partially be an unintended consequence of the purging combined with her other healthy lifestyle practices. The imbalance of avalambaka kapha correlates with the mild imbalances in the heart and pericardium. Their mildness expresses the resilience of her youth but looming issues in the future.

Naturally, her upper digestive tract will be completely imbalanced due to the repetitive unnatural use of the functions of vata. This explains the imbalance in the rasa dhatu. The imbalance in the asthi dhatu was being expressed because of Mandy's dental health. After Mandy's revelation, the pulse reader made sure to examine her teeth, which were stripped of their protective linings by the excess exposure to the acidity from purging. The inherent leaning towards the excessive utilization of rajas correlates to the extreme anxiety Mandy experiences leading to her behavior. The presence of tamas in the second layer is the result of that excess activity over the years creating ups and downs that are mirrored in the binging and purging behavior. Her overall agni and dhatu agnis are depleted to the point that they cannot produce the essences of prana, tejas and ojas.

MANDY'S SAMPRAPTI

In the case of Mandy, the samprapti is as follows:

1. Excessive utilization of rajas drives Mandy to partake in lifestyle behaviors that cause all three doshas to *accumulate* in their respective seats. Vata, in the colon, pitta in the small intestine, and kapha in the stomach.

2. Mandy *provokes* all three accumulated doshas by binging and purging. Kapha is provoked mainly through binging, pitta is provoked by both binging and purging, and vata is provoked by both binging and purging.

3. The three doshas *spread* throughout the body in their agitated form while functioning abnormally. Mandy's gastrointestinal tract begins to function abnormally and her acid reflux begins.

4. The improperly functioning doshas then *localize* in the various dhatus and organs, negatively affecting their generation, regeneration and function. Mandy's gallbladder begins to fail, her pericardium and heart experience strain and her teeth begin to lose their protective linings.

5. Upon localizing in various dhatus, the doshas begin to *manifest* their qualities in an unnatural manner, physically altering the structure and formation of the dhatus. Mandy's depletion sets in and the dhatus begin to change their form throughout her entire body.

6. If the root cause continues, ultimately the manifestation *differentiates* into multiple, self-contained pathologies. While Mandy was not experiencing this stage in its fullness, she could very well develop a myriad of conditions later on that would not necessarily be resolved by the cessation of the root cause.

The pulse reader, assimilating all of this, now has a new understanding of how behaviors such as these are expressed by the pulse and will carry that wisdom into future pulse readings.

EXAMPLE OF A COMPLETE PULSE READING "RAY"

Sex: Male
Age: 52
Height: 5'10"
Weight: 165lbs
Occupation: Restaurant Owner
Relationship Status: Single, Divorced
Children: One
Appointment Time: 2:00pm

Ray's primary complaints are lower and middle back pain, mild memory loss, low libido, lack of appetite and constipation. Upon walking into the room, the pulse reader suspects that he has a pitta-vata prominent prakruti based on his bone structure and facial features. After a brief introduction and conversation regarding his reasons for coming, the pulse reader requests Ray' right wrist. He casually offers his wrist while commenting that he just had his pulses read at his doctor's office last week. The pulse reader takes this opportunity to explain that ayurvedic pulse reading is a little different, that he can close his eyes and relax as it will take a few minutes.

Ray nods his head and closes his eyes, squirming around in his chair until he finds a comfortable position. Shortly after Ray settles in, he needs to move again to adjust his back. His wrist jerks each time. The pulse reader can easily see that Ray is quite uncomfortable and his movements will be distracting to the pulse reading. The pulse reader asks Ray if he would be more comfortable laying down. Ray says he would, and they move into the therapy room so that Ray can lay on a massage table on his back while the pulse reader sits in a chair to perform the reading. Ray lets out a sigh, his body much more relaxed.

RAY'S PULSES

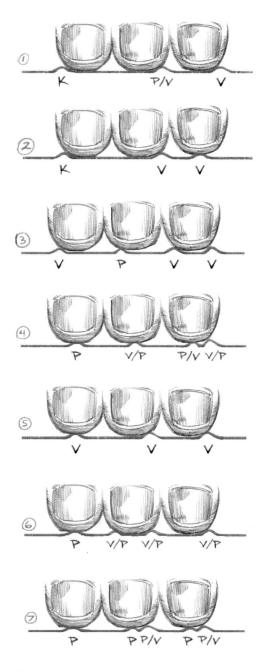

Image 76 - Ray's Pulses

Before the pulse reader takes Ray's right wrist, she or he remembers that it is 2pm, both the pulse reader and likely Ray have eaten not too long ago. This would influence the expression of his pulses towards kapha, as would laying on his back. The pulse reader asks Ray if he ate lunch before the appointment. Ray says no, that he usually skips lunch because that is one of his busiest times at the restaurant. The pulse reader takes note of his off tempo eating schedule.

Placing the fingertips on Ray's right wrist on the vikruti layer of the pulse, the pulse reader immediately experiences the expression of both vata and kapha qualities and Ray's warm, dry skin. Before assessing this layer further, the pulse reader delves to the prakruti layer.

The seventh layer confirms the suspected prakruti. The ring finger crest makes contact on the pitta location. The middle and index fingers are each contacted by two crests. The crests make contact with the fingertips on both the pitta and vata locations. The qualities expressed in the crests are consistently sharp and forceful. The rate is quick, about 78 beats per minute. The gait feels like the pulse is jumping suggesting a pitta nature. The force is ample also suggesting a pitta nature. The volume is slightly narrow, expressing a vata nature. The texture and quality of the artery itself is a little tough and resistant, suggesting a vata nature due to a lesser proportion of kapha in the tissue. The surface temperature of the skin is warm, suggesting a pitta nature.

The rhythm is steady overall but seems to change slightly each time Ray breathes. To confirm this, the pulse reader checks for a respiratory sinus arrhythmia. The pulse reader asks Ray to take a deep breath, hold it briefly, and then exhale completely. There is a clearly discernable change in his pulse rate of approximately three beats per minute.

The pulse reader surfaces to the vikruti layer to assess it more thoroughly. The ring fingertip is contacted by a crest at the kapha location and is expressing kapha qualities. It is of medium breadth and feels dull, not exerting much force against the fingertip. It is not in alignment with the prakruti layer ring finger crest in either location or quality. The middle fingertip is contacted by a crest on the vata location. It is expressing both pitta and vata qualities, only slightly narrow, lightly touching the fingertip but with clear definition. It is similar to the prakruti expression but leans more on the side of vata expression and lacks the fullness of the prakruti pulse's pitta expression. The index fingertip is contacted at the vata location. It is expressing the vata qualities and feels narrow, stringy, ephemeral and light. It mirrors the prakruti layer only in the location of the vata crest location. The pulse reader notes that while there is certainly some alignment with the prakruti pulse expression, there is an overall lack of pitta expression in both location and quality. The kapha crest expressing kapha qualities on the ring fingertip stands out as well. The pulse reader delves back to the seventh layer for reference, and then ascends to the sixth layer of the pulse.

Overall, the sixth layer of the pulse feels similar in quality to the seventh layer. The force and breadth feel consistent with the seventh layer findings. The ring fingertip is contacted by a crest on the pitta location. It matches the prakruti pulse is both location and quality expressing that Ray's mind has a level of inclination towards sattva. The middle fingertip is contacted by a crest on both the kapha and vata locations. Both crests are expressing the vata quality of pin-pointedness at the location of contact but with a moderate amount of force. The pulse reader discerns that while the vata crest matches the prakruti expression, the quality and presence of the kapha crest do not convey sattvic leanings, but rather rajasic and potentially tamasic leanings. The index fingertip is contacted by a crest at the vata location. It is similar in location and quality to the vata crest on the prakruti layer but feels subtly "off." There is also no presence of a pitta crest to match the prakruti expression. Again, the pulse reader discerns that there may be a sattvic leaning of the mind, but also senses a rajasic leaning. Overall, Ray's mind appears to inherently utilize rajas but not without the presence of sattvic influence. Taking note of all this, the pulse reader ascends to the first layer for reference, and then delves into the second layer.

The second layer of the pulse tells a slightly different story than the sixth layer. The kapha crest on the ring fingertip is expressing kapha qualities, similar to the vikruti layer. The pulse reader recognizes that this was the crest that expressed the clearest connection with the mind's sattvic leanings on the sixth layer. It is now expressing more tamasic activity. The middle fingertip is contacted by a crest in the vata location expressing vata qualities feeling thread-like. Unlike the sixth layer, there is no presence of a crest at the kapha location. The index finger is contacted by a crest at the pitta location and is expressing the same thread-like vata quality. It also differs from the sixth layer expression. While both the middle fingertip and index fingertip are contacted by crests that mirror, in part, the expression of the prakruti pulse, the pulse reader is hesitant to interpret them as indication of sattvic mental activity. There is too much dissonance overall between location and qualities, and the presence of the tamas expressing itself through the ring fingertip solidifies this. The pulse reader feels that these are more likely expressions of rajas and that Ray has lost touch with his sattvic leanings at this present moment. From here, the pulse reader delves to the third layer.

On the third layer of the pulse the ring fingertip crest is making contact at the tarpaka kapha location. It is expressing the vata quality of a pinprick and feels feeble. The pulse reader immediately connects this to Ray's complaint of some mild memory loss. The middle fingertip crest is making contact at the location of alochaka pitta. It feels relatively full and moderately forceful and has a similarity in quality to the overall expression of the prakruti. The pulse reader moves on to the index finger which is being contacted by a crest at the apana vata location and the prana vata location. Both crests are expressing vata qualities quite prominently. They are feeble, light and narrow. The pulse reader takes note of the correlation between imbalanced prana vata and tarpaka kapha as well as remembering Ray's complaint regarding intermittent constipation which relates to apana vata. The presence of imbalanced prana vata activity in the context of imbalanced apana vata gives the pulse reader the confidence to make a link between the tendencies towards constipation and an imbalance in the brain tissue, primarily composed of majja dhatu and largely governed by tarpaka kapha.

While the activity of alochaka pitta did not feel imbalanced at this time, the pulse reader also takes note of the proximity of the eyes to one of the primary sites of imbalance. At this point, the pulse reader delves past the fourth layer and into the fifth layer.

The crest on the ring fingertip is making contact at the location expressing shukra dhatu. It is very feeble and thread-like in feeling. The crest on the middle fingertip is making contact at the location of meda dhatu. It is also very feeble and thread-like in feeling. The crest on the index fingertip is making contact at the majja dhatu location. It feels like a soft tapping against the very edge of the fingertip and almost seems to touch the fingertip twice before diffusing, expressing an unnatural and highly vata aggravated gait. The pulse reader immediately makes the connection between the majja dhatu and what was experienced on the third layer of the pulse. The weakness of the shukra dhatu expression is confirming of this. The inherent connection between the meda dhatu and the majja dhatu dawns on the pulse reader. If the meda dhatu is depleted, the majja dhatu is likely to be as well. Ray's complaints of back pain, low libido, memory loss and constipation as well as the eyes' relationship with majja dhatu are all coming together within the expression of the pulse. With this knowledge, the pulse reader ascends to the fourth and final layer.

The fourth layer of the pulse expresses and overall feeling of moderate breadth and force, similar to the prakruti. The pervading presence of vata qualities, while not completely absent, are certainly less prominent. Each of the crests on all three fingertips are making contact at the location of tejas. There is an additional crest making contact at the location of prana on the index fingertip. This almost mirrors the prakruti exactly with the exception of a missing crest on the prana location of the middle fingertip. At first, the pulse reader is not quite sure what to make of this level of balance on the fourth layer in the context of the other layers. Taking a breath, the pulse reader re-focuses on each of the fingertips again. Upon doing so the pulse reader picks up on two subtleties that went unnoticed. The first is the presence of the same imbalanced gait on the prana crest of the index finger. The second is a slightly hollow feeling expressed by the crest on the middle fingertip. This information is enough to aid the pulse reader in perceiving a lack of the presence of ojas on this layer. It is clear that Ray utilizes tejas heavily. He is dressed well, has a charming personality, owns and operates his own business and is clearly extroverted. In the context of all the other layers, the pulse reader discerns that Ray is utilizing tejas disproportionately to the amount of ojas his prakruti naturally generates and is currently available in his body. In Ray's younger years this would have likely gone completely unnoticed. As vata slowly destabilized through his life, his outward activity began to outrun his inward nourishment. With this in mind, and all the layers read, the pulse reader moves on to assess the organ pulses.

RAY'S ORGAN PULSES

LEFT RADIAL ARTERY			RIGHT RADIAL ARTERY		
ORGAN	CREST LOCATION	QUALITY	ORGAN	CREST LOCATION	QUALITY
SMALL INTESTINE	PITTA	PITTA	COLON	VATA	VATA
HEART	PITTA	PITTA	LUNGS	PITTA	VATA
STOMACH	VATA	VATA	GALLBLADDER	PITTA	PITTA
SPLEEN & PANCREAS	VATA	VATA	LIVER	KAPHA	PITTA/KAPHA
BLADDER	PITTA	PITTA/KAPHA	PERICARDIUM	PITTA	PITTA
KIDNEYS	PITTA	PITTA/KAPHA	CIRCULATION	VATA	PITTA

The pulse reader places the index finger alone on the first layer of Ray's right radial artery correlating to the colon. As suspected, the crest makes contact with the fingertip on the vata location and is expressing feeble, narrow qualities. The pulse reader delves down to the seventh layer to read the pulse correlating to the lungs. The crest is making contact at the pitta location and is mildly expressing the vata qualities of lightness and narrowness.

The pulse reader replaces the index finger with the middle finger and places it on the first layer of the radial artery to assess the pulse correlating with the gallbladder. The crest is making contact at the pitta location. The pulse is full and of medium breadth, mirroring the qualities found in the prakruti expression. The pulse reader delves to the seventh layer to read the pulse correlating to the liver. The crest is making contact at the kapha location. It is also of medium breadth and applying a medium amount of force. However, the pulse reader notices that it feels slightly dull as though the crest is blunted at the point of contact, expressing a mild kapha imbalance given Ray's prakruti and the nature of the liver as heavily pitta prominent organ.

The pulse reader replaces the middle finger with the ring finger to assess the first layer pulse correlating to the pericardium. The crest is making contact at the pitta location and feels relatively balanced. The pulse reader delves to the seventh layer to assess the pulse correlating to circulation. The crest makes contact at the vata location and is expressing the pitta qualities of forcefulness and sharpness. The pulse reader makes the connection to constipation, the deterioration of tarpaka kapha, and Ray's high velocity lifestyle. This pattern could indicate future circulatory issues including hypertension and, more dramatically, stroke.

Before completely disengaging from Ray's right wrist the pulse reader requests Ray's left hand to read both pulses simultaneously. The pulse reader notices that overall, Ray's right radial artery is expressing with more force and breadth than the left. The difference is noticeable, but not terribly dramatic. It is confirming of Ray's overexertion and inclination to operate within his sympathetic nervous system.

Moving to the left wrist, the pulse reader briefly checks in on the prakruti layer and the vikruti layer to see if they mirror the right pulse. They are expressing themselves similarly, so the pulse reader moves on to read the organs associated with the left radial artery.

Placing only the index finger on the left radial artery, the pulse reader assesses the pulse correlating to the small intestine. The crest is contacting the fingertip in the pitta location. The pitta qualities feel slightly excessive. The bounding pulse is pushing quite forcefully against the index fingertip. The pulse reader delves to the seventh layer to perceive the pulse correlated with the heart. It feels very similar to the small intestine pulse and makes contact on the same location of the fingertip. Pitta appears to be provoked and potentially spreading throughout the body.

The index finger is replaced by the middle finger which the pulse reader places on the first layer corresponding to the stomach. The crest is making contact on the vata location. The pulse is mildly feeble but relatively broad. The pulse reader notices a slight quiver at the peak of the crest suggesting a variable and slightly unstable agni. The pulse reader remembers that Ray's eating schedule is erratic and most likely has been for some time. Delving to the seventh layer, the pulse reader assesses the pulse correlating to the spleen and pancreas. It feels very similar to the pulse expressing the state of the stomach reconfirming Ray's temperamental agni, especially given the pancreas' role in digestion.

The pulse reader removes the middle finger and places the ring finger on the first layer pulse corresponding to the bladder. The crest makes contact with the fingertip on the pitta location and carries mainly pitta qualities but with blunted expression at the peak of the crest. Upon delving to the seventh layer correlating to the kidneys, the pulse reader finds the same expression likely revealing some degree of ama. The pulse reader also suspects that this is related to the imbalanced functioning of apana vata, but that the colon is affected more severely.

The pulse reader takes a breath and removes her or his hand from Ray's wrist. After a brief pause, the pulse reader decides to check Ray's navel pulse since he is already laying on the massage table. Requesting that Ray take a few deep breaths, the pulse reader plunges all five fingers into the umbilicus on Ray's exhale while he is instructed to hold his breath out momentarily. The navel pulse is powerful and steady but not centered. Though the pulse reader's fingers are located directly at the center of the umbilicus, he or she can feel the pulse resonating approximately an inch higher and to the right. This serves as further confirmation that the subdoshas of vata, especially samana vata and apana vata are imbalanced. It also gives the pulse reader a good indication of Ray's current stress and anxiety levels.

DISCUSSING THE FINDINGS

When Ray gets up from the massage table, he takes a moment to stretch his back and roll his shoulders. The sounds of cracking joints are audible. They return to the office to discuss the findings. While *confident* in the overall reading, the pulse reader recognizes that he or she is not completely *neutral.* Something about Ray reminds the pulse reader of a previous employer with whom the pulse reader did not completely get along. Keeping this in mind the pulse reader continues, acknowledging the bias but allowing the *compassion* for Ray's situation to take priority. The pulse reader is aware that Ray has little to no experience with ayurveda. As such, the pulse reader decides to be extremely simplistic in the explanation of the findings for the sake of *clarity.*

Through all the findings, the pulse reader senses that the imbalance in apana vata is of the utmost importance.

From this insight, the pulse reader begins to discuss the findings intentionally starting with constipation and its probable connection to his low libido and back pain. The pulse reader *discerns* Ray's discomfort around the subject though it is hidden behind a smile. Pausing, the pulse reader asks Ray if he has any question so far. Ray shakes his head slowly. He explains that the doesn't have a question, but he would like to discuss something very private. The pulse reader assures Ray that everything that is discussed in the session is held in strict confidence.

Ray expresses that after his divorce, when he was in his late 30's, he developed what he deems an addiction to sex and masturbation, ejaculating sometimes more than thirty times in a month. In his late 40's he slowed down because he felt drained and needed to keep up his energy to run his restaurant which was experiencing hard times. His constipation began shortly after the divorce as well, which he believes was due to the erratic diet he developed in his vacillations between loneliness and short-term relationships. He also reduced his sexual activity because he was starting to have erectile difficulties and ejaculating prematurely. He didn't want to deal with the embarrassment he experienced around his sex life, so he stopped seeking partnership completely.

The pulse reader thanks Ray for disclosing all of this and they begin a dialogue on the importance of shukra dhatu and apana vata in a manner that Ray finds accessible. The pulse reader explains how all of his symptoms are connected to the repeated, long-term depletion of shukra dhatu, which in turn, compromises the robustness of all the dhatus, especially majja dhatu, which is driving his memory loss.

In addition to a number of lifestyle and dietary changes, the pulse reader suggests that Ray undergo panchakarma to halt the progression of his imbalance, begin the long process of rejuvenating his depleted shukra and majja dhatus, and potentially reverse the pathology altogether.

After Ray leaves, the pulse reader reviews the findings for his or her own benefit. The imbalance in apana vata was being driven by Ray's excessive sexual activity. From there the other issues developed from the back pain to the memory loss. Ray was prone to this type of behavior imbalance from the excess utilization of rajas throughout his life. While Ray's sixth layer pulse indicated a sattvic leaning of the mind, during the session Ray explained that in the years leading up to his divorce he felt like he had "lost himself" to some degree, likely marking the transition towards a fully tamas and rajas driven lifestyle. Ray's desire to seek holistic aid is an opportunity for him to recultivate his sattvic inclinations, which will help him uphold a more healthful lifestyle.

In the case of Ray, the samprapti is as follows:

1. Excess utilization of rajas drives Ray to engage in lifestyle behaviors that result in the *accumulation* of vata in the bladder, kidneys, and primarily the colon.
2. Ray increases the behaviors that caused the accumulation of apana vata, *provoking* not only apana vata, but vata in general. This begins to influence the pitta dosha in the upper

gastrointestinal tract as well.

3. Continuation of the behaviors over time encourages the *spread* of vata throughout the body. Secondarily, pitta begins to spread as well, though not as dramatically.

4. The aggravated vata dosha *localizes* in the meda and majja dhatus. These dhatus were already susceptible because of Ray's health history. Since Ray's prakruti is not kapha prominent, it does not inherently guard against the negative influences of aggravated vata.

5. The localization of vata eventually *manifests* as the symptoms of back pain, erectile disfunction, premature ejaculation, depletion of protective joint fluid linings, and memory loss. All of these symptoms reflect the altered structure and function of the relevant dhatus.

6. Ray's memory loss is likely the first sign of *differentiation*. If it were to progress it would not necessarily subside merely from the cessation of the root causes. If Ray were to experience a stroke in the future, any damage to his dhatus from the event would also exemplify *differentiation*.

The pulse reader, assimilating all of this, now has a new understanding of how behaviors such as these are expressed by the pulse and will carry that wisdom into future pulse readings.

OVERALL

Both the cases of Mandy and Ray present hidden lifestyle components that are major contributing factors to the underlying imbalances. They are not readily shared as they are quite vulnerable for rogis to express. This is more often the case then not. Without addressing these, little healing will take place. The pulse reader not only utilizes the reading to express the findings, but also creates opportunities for the rogi to express deeper vulnerabilities by choosing when and how to unveil specific findings.

CHAPTER SEVENTEEN

PULSE READING BEYOND HUMANS – DOGS, CATS AND HORSES

A FEW WORDS ON CAUTION

Not all animals are comfortable having their pulses read. Do <u>not</u> read an unfamiliar animal's pulse unless professionally trained to do so. Even with familiar animals, if the animal shows any signs of discomfort, agitation or aggression then cease immediately. Do <u>not</u> close your eyes while reading an animal's pulse. Visually monitor the animal's body language and signaling at all times.

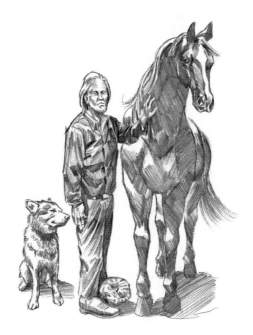

Image 77 - Dog, Cat and Horse

Any living being with a heart has a pulse, and that pulse expresses the entirety of its essence and form with each beat.

The principles of Ayurveda are the principles of Nature. As such, they encompass all living beings. As far as the practice of pulse reading is concerned, it is primarily used to assess dogs, cats and horses.

DOGS AND CATS

The primary site for reading the pulse of a dog or cat is the femoral artery. The femoral artery is located on the inside of the hind legs and runs down the thigh to the lower leg. It is most easily read on the inside of the thigh close to the abdomen.

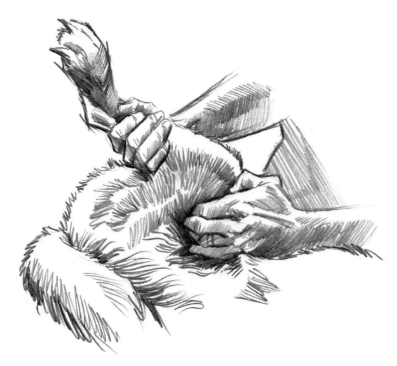

Image 78 - Dog's Femoral Artery

The pulse reader utilizes the same three fingers she or he does to read a human's pulse. The ring finger is placed closest to the abdomen,

173

and thus the heart, while the index finger is closest to the paw. It is much more difficult to read the layers of a dog or cat's pulse for a few reasons. The first is the unlikelihood that the dog or cat will remain still long enough to engage in the subtle detection of layered pulse reading. Second is that unlike the radial artery of a human, there is no clear reference or solid surface defining the bottom layer. If the dog or cat is very calm, the pulse reader may attempt to read a deep layer communicating the prakruti, and a shallow layer communicating the vikruti.

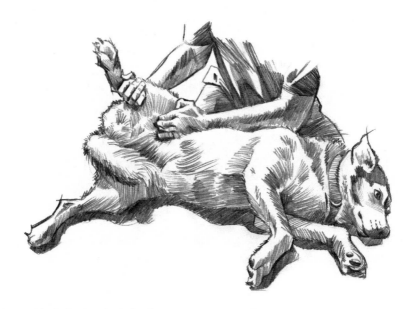

Image 79 - Pulse Reader Behind Dog

The dog or cat can be standing or on its side while the pulse reader reaches underneath its hind leg, <u>*not*</u> from between its tail and leg but from between its leg and abdomen. The pulse reader may gently grip the leg with the alternate hand, stabilizing the dog or cat in the proper position.

The principles of reading a human's pulse are largely the same as when reading a dog or cat's pulse. There are a few key differences. Dogs and cats have a faster heart rate in general. Small dogs have heart rates of 120 to 160 beats per minute. Medium sized dogs over

30 pounds have heart rates of 80 to 120 beats per minute. Cats have heart rates that range from 140 to 220 beats per minute. The breadth of the femoral artery is larger than that of the radial artery. This does not mean that dogs and cats are more kapha in nature than humans. It is simply due to the size of the artery.

The prakruti and vikruti of a dog or cat must be determined in the context of both the breed as a whole and within the breed itself. For example, the Saint Bernard breed as a whole is kapha prominent. There are vata, pitta and kapha prominent Saint Bernards relative to each other. The chihuahua breed as a whole is vata dominant but there are vata, pitta, and kapha prominent chihuahuas relative to each other.

HORSES

The primary site for reading a horse's pulse is on the digital artery of the legs. It is located above the hoof and on the side of the pastern. It can be slightly difficult to locate. The pulse reader's ring finger is placed closest to the pastern, and thus the heart, and the index finger is closest to the hoof.

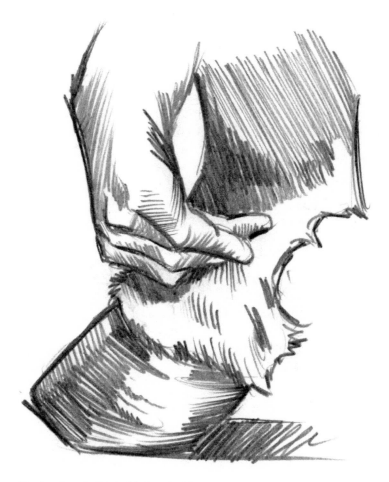

Image 80 - Reading the Digital Pulse of a Horse

Horses, being much larger animals, have an average heart rate of 32 to 36 beats per minute. The prakruti and vikruti of a horse is read in the same manner as with dogs and cats. The breed as a whole tends towards a type of prakruti and then individuals within the breed express all three vata, pitta and kapha prominences. For example, thoroughbreds as a breed are more pitta prominent while Clydesdales are more kapha prominent.

CHAPTER EIGHTEEN

PRACTICES TO ENHANCE PULSE READING

Both the sense of hearing and touch, with their corresponding mental unions as listening and feeling, are governed by vata. As such the pulse reader's overall capacity to clearly and accurately perceive the pulse rests on the balanced state of vata in the pulse reader's body.

Following the wisdom of Ayurveda as a whole is one of the most effective ways to enhance the pulse reader's capacities. It encourages the cultivation of sattva, balances the doshas, balances and strengthens all the dhatus, keeps the organs functioning at peak performance and prepares the body for spiritual experiences allowing deeper access to intuition. Beyond a sattvic diet, daily routine and seasonal routine there are a few well known practices with a particular affinity to the art of pulse reading. Pranayama, mudra and mantra are powerful tools in developing one's own mind, consciousness, and autonomic nervous system. There are many practices that a pulse reader can adopt to improve. Below are but a few.

SHEETALI PRANAYAMA

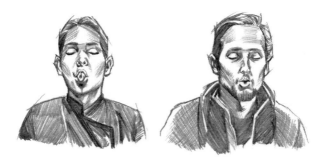

Image 81 - Two Versions of Sheetali Pranayama

Sheetali means cold. This pranayama not only cools the body but also nervous system activity so that the pulse reader can become calm and quiet in his or her internal experience of the mind. The ability to transition from highly active to calm relatively quickly is an absolute crucial skill for the pulse reader to develop. This does not simply mean thinking the thought, "be calm," but entails that the pulse reader enter deeply into the parasympathetic nervous system prior to reading the pulse. The breath is invaluable in this transition. The daily practice of this pranayama engrains a deep sense of calm in the practitioner. From this state, the pulse reader can be neutral minded and sattvic in attitude.

There are two ways to perform sheetali pranayama. In both versions the eyes are closed. The first is with the tongue curled into a "U" shape, sticking out of the mouth. The practitioner inhales deeply into the abdomen as slowly as possible through the tongue. The air will feel cool or cold entering the body. The tongue is then put back into the mouth and the practitioner exhales through the nose drawing the exhale out as long as possible. This process is then repeated.

Not everyone can curl the tongue into a "U" shape. In lieu of this the practitioner can pucker his or her lips into an "O" shape and drink the air as if through a straw. The same effect of cool or cold air running over the tongue and into the body is achieved. The practitioner then closes her or his mouth and exhales through the nose as deeply and for as long as possible. This breath can be performed eleven to twenty-six repetitions daily.

In some cases, the practitioner may notice a bitter taste on the sides of the tongue. This is a sign that the liver is detoxifying, releasing ama into the bloodstream to be evacuated. This exercise should be avoided if the practitioner has a very low heart rate, low blood pressure or chronic cardiac issues.

HAKINI MUDRA

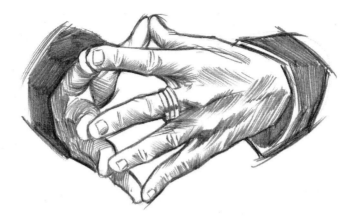

Image 82 - Hakini Mudra

In this mudra the five fingertips come together at diaphragm level, the fingertips pointing away from the body. They are spread apart forming a pyramid-like shape. There are versions of this mudra in which the fingers are slightly rounded as if holding a sphere.

Hakini mudra is named after the Hindu goddess Hakini. She is the personification of the ajna chakra, the third eye, which correlates to the pituitary gland physiologically. This is the seat of intuition and holding this mudra aids in opening the channels that allow the intuition to flourish. Mudras such as this one must be practiced regularly, preferably daily, to obtain their intended effect.

This mudra can be held for any length of time, but eleven to thirty-one minutes is long enough to experience its effects. With practice, the pulse reader should be able to feel pulsations between all ten fingertips. This is an indication that the circulation to the fingertips is very strong and the dhatus contained in the fingertips are receiving an abundance of nourishment. It encourages new nerve pathways and connections to form in the fingertips, increasing their capacity to receive and perceive information transferred through touch.

Hakini mudra also benefits short-term and long-term memory by balancing tarpaka kapha. The short-term memory improvement is

179

especially useful for the pulse reader as he or she needs to remember the crest locations and qualities on each layer of the pulse during the reading. It also balances blood pressure which contributes to the pulse reader's sense of overall wellbeing and calmness.

SUNIA

Chanting mantra, creating a repetitive sound current with which the mind can become absorbed, is the third crucial tool a pulse reader can utilize. There are thousands of mantras available, all with different effects and for different circumstances. Chanting in general moves the body into a parasympathetic state and encourages the mind to tranquilly reside in its seat, the heart.

Every spiritual tradition identifies the importance of sunia. Sunia, pronounced suni-ai, means deep, complete, listening. The kind of listening in which the individual feels empty and receptive. The kind of listening necessary for sophisticated, intuitive and subtle pulse reading. Below is one version of a sunia mantra. This version is from the Sikh tradition of Northern India. It can be repeated eleven, fifty-four or 108 times in a sitting.

ਸੁਣਿਐ ਸਤੁ ਸੰਤੋਖੁ ਗਿਆਨੁ ॥
ਸੁਣਿਐ ਅਠਸਠਿ ਕਾ ਇਸਨਾਨੁ ॥
ਸੁਣਿਐ ਪੜਿ ਪੜਿ ਪਾਵਹਿ ਮਾਨੁ ॥
ਸੁਣਿਐ ਲਾਗੈ ਸਹਜਿ ਧਿਆਨੁ ॥
ਨਾਨਕ ਭਗਤਾ ਸਦਾ ਵਿਗਾਸੁ ॥
ਸੁਣਿਐ ਦੂਖ ਪਾਪ ਕਾ ਨਾਸੁ ॥੧੦॥

SUNI-AI SAT SANTOKH GIAAN

SUNI-AI ATHSATH KAA ISANAAN

SUNI-AI PAR PAR PAAVEH MAAN

SUNI-AI LAGAI SAHAJ DHI-AAN

NAANAK BHAGATAA SADAA VIGAAS

SUNI-AI DOOKH PAAP KAA NAAS

Listening and absorbing the holy teachings, brings truthfulness, offerings, contentment and spiritual illumination.

Listening and absorbing the holy teachings is equal in blessings to bathing at the sixty-eight places of pilgrimage.

By listening and absorbing the holy teachings, people have received honor through their studies.

By listening and absorbing the holy teachings, the mind is cooled in meditation.

Nanak, God's devotees are always in bliss.

By listening and absorbing the holy teachings, they are released from suffering and pain.

FINAL WORDS

As the pulse reader practices the techniques described, he or she will begin to develop a unique kind of sense. Patterns will emerge, insights will present themselves. The structure with which the pulse reader begins will become more fluid, as the pulse reader's confidence increases. The confidence of the pulse reader increases with each connection made in which the pulse reader receives confirmation of its truth. The pulse reader's self-talk will become clearer, simpler, and more direct. All of this unfolds with repetition and reading a wide variety of pulses.

With experience, the pulse reader will develop his or her own nuances when reading the pulse. Pulse reading is a communication between two highly sophisticated living beings, and its subtleties are endless. Pulse readers should not be afraid to explore perceived patterns and their correlations in the body, regardless of whether they are referenced in a text or have been discussed by great pulse readers of the past.

The art of pulse reading offers the student opportunities to go beyond his or her common perception of the world. There are pulse readers who practice an art known as doot nadi. This practice involves reading the pulse of the messenger who delivers news of the status of a rogi. By assessing the messenger's pulse, the pulse reader ascertains the condition of the rogi. Such practices require that the pulse reader perceive the more subtle realms of experience and energies at play. To do so requires the release of what has now become the conventional understanding of how the world works. Pulse reading's expansive and subtle reach is part of the beauty of the art.

Above all, be patient. It takes a great deal of practice to cultivate one's own pulse reading capacities. Some believe that the skill of pulse reading is developed over many lifetimes.

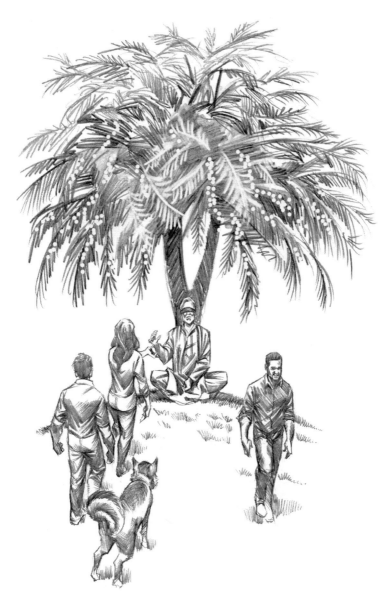

Image 83 - Master Pulse Reader Under an Amla Tree

GLOSSARY

<u>A</u>

Acharya - One who perceives patterns.

Akash - Sanskrit word meaning "ether." In the context of Ayurveda the primary quality of ether is spaciousness.

Alochaka Pitta - A subdosha of pitta located in the eyes and responsible for sight.

Agni - Sanskrit word meaning "fire." It is also used in the context of Ayurveda to describe the body's ability to transform nourishment into tissues and doshas.

Ahara - Anything that nourishes the body. This can include foods, liquids and sense perceptions.

Amla Tree - Phyllanthus emblica. Also known and Indian gooseberry. The fruit from this tree is a renown ayurvedic remedy. The Sanskrit word 'amla' means sour. Amla fruit is primarily sour in taste. It has one of the richest sources of vitamin 'C' in the world.

Apana Vata - A subdosha of vata governing the downward and outward movements in the body.

Arthava - A "sub dhatu" of shukra dhatu. It is found only in women and comprises the tissues and organs involved in menstruation

Asthi Dhatu - The constituent of bone tissue.

Autonomic Nervous System - Part of the central nervous system. The autonomic nervous system regulates most of the automatic functions in the body such as heart rate and unconscious breathing. The autonomic nervous system is comprised of the parasympathetic and sympathetic nervous systems.

Avalambaka Kapha - A subdosha of kapha primarily enveloping and protecting the heart and lungs. It acts as a cushion against the constant movement of the heart and lungs.

Ayurveda - The science of life

184

B

Bulimia, Binging and Purging - An eating disorder defined by the act of eating large quantities of food quickly after denying one's self for a period of time. Vomiting is then forcefully induced to remove the food from the stomach before it is assimilated by the body.

Bhrajaka Pitta - A subdosha of pitta located in the skin. It is responsible for regulating the temperature of the body as well as transdermal nourishment and evacuation.

Bodhaka Kapha - A subdosha of kapha located in the mouth. It is responsible for the sense of taste and begins the digestive process with saliva.

C

Carotid Artery - The major artery in the neck on either side of the jugular.

Clarity - A quality of character that allows the pulse reader to express the findings of a pulse reading in a way that the rogi can understand.

Compassion - A quality of character that allows the pulse reader to understand what a rogi needs to heal above all else.

Confidence - A quality of character that allows the pulse reader to believe in what he or she finds in the pulses. Confidence in the context of pulse reading is based on experience and intuition.

Crest – The basic form of a pulse wave as it makes contact with a fingertip.

D

Darshana - In the context of Ayurveda, darshana refers to the pulse reader's use of vision to assist in the diagnosis of a rogi's condition.

Dhatu - A major tissue of the body. There are seven in total.

Digital Artery - A location in which a pulse reader can find the pulse of a horse. It is located above the hoof, on the side of the pastern.

Discernment - A quality of character that allows the pulse reader to perceive what course of action will be most helpful to a rogi at any given moment.

Doot Nadi - The practice of reading the pulse of the messenger in order to assess the condition of the rogi

Dosha - A Sanskrit word meaning "that which falls out of balance." It refers to vata, pitta and kapha. The three doshas harmonize to perform the biological functions in the body and the whole of nature. Each dosha is composed of two elements and each dosha carries unique, qualities that determine its functions.

E

Element - There are five elements called the "pancha mahabhutas" in Sanskrit. They are akash, vayu, agni, jala and prithvi. They form the basic components of everything in the physical world. Each possess unique qualities from which it is inseparable.

F

Femoral Artery - A major artery running from the inside of the thigh down the leg. It can be used to assess the pulse in humans, dogs and cats.

Force - In the context of pulse reading, force refers to the amount of pressure blood exerts on the vessel wall with each heartbeat.

G

Gait - In the context of pulse reading, gait refers to the movement of a crest across a portion of the fingertip. The gait can be regular or irregular depending on the state of balance or imbalance within the body.

Guna - The mental qualities of sattva, rajas and tamas.

H

Hakini Mudra - Named after the goddess Hakini, this mudra consists of placing all ten fingertips together at diaphragm level. It benefits the pituitary gland, which correlates to intuition.

I

Ida - The feminine, lunar channel. It begins on the left side of the body at the base of the spine and crisscrosses with the pingala and sushumna, through all of the chakras terminating in the sixth chakra at the brow point. It corresponds with the functions of the parasympathetic nervous system.

Intuition - The pulse reader's capacity to synthesize sophisticated and subtle information beyond rational understanding.

J

Jala – Sanskrit word meaning "water." In the context of Ayurveda the primary quality of jala is fluidity.

K

Kapha - One of the three primary doshas. Kapha is composed of jala and prithvi. It forms containers and protective linings in the body.

Kledaka Kapha - A subdosha of kapha located in the stomach. It protects the stomach from the hydrochloric acid the stomach secretes. It also combines with food in the stomach to prevent the food from overexposure to acidity, which would destroy the nourishment.

L

Lifestyle – In an ayurvedic context lifestyle refers to all of the behaviors one carries out on a daily basis that contribute to either the balance or imbalance of his or her body and mind.

M

Majja - One of the seven dhatus. It is found inside large bones. Majja is the constituent of bone marrow, nerves, and cerebrospinal fluid.

Mala - The bi-product of the creation of a dhatu. Malas are either evacuated or reused within the body.

Mamsa - One of the seven dhatus. Mamsa is the constituent that forms muscle fibers.

Mantra - A specific word or phrase to be used repetitively, often in the form of a chant, to create a specific effect.

Meda - One of the seven dhatus. It is the constituent that forms adipose tissue.

Mudra - A specific hand posture to be held in order to create a certain effect.

N

Nadi Pariksha - Sanskrit for "pulse reading."

Nadi Vijnana - Sanskrit for "pulse diagnosis"

Neutrality - A quality of character that allows the pulse reader to remain non-reactive in the face of personal biases in order to perceive the pulse accurately. It is necessary for discernment.

O

Ojas - A highly refined form of kapha that creates resilience. Ojas is created by contributions from all of the dhatus. The body requires it to survive. It is also necessary for the proper functioning of the immune system. The most refined form of ojas resides in the heart.

P

Pachaka Pitta - A subdosha of pitta located in digestive fluids. Pachaka pitta breaks down food into its basic elements to be used by the dhatu agnis to form dhatus. Its seat is in the stomach.

Parasympathetic Nervous System - Part of the autonomic nervous system. The parasympathetic nervous system engages the body's restorative, digestive and reproductive functions.

Pingala - The masculine, solar channel. It begins on the right side of the body at the base of the spine and crisscrosses with the ida and sushumna, through all of the chakras terminating in the sixth chakra at the brow point. It corresponds with the functions of the sympathetic nervous system.

Pitta - One of the three primary doshas. Pitta is composed of agni and jala. It governs the transformation of nourishment into dhatus. It is responsible for the proper functioning of the metabolism.

Prakruti - The basic, unchangeable, balanced, constitution unique to each living being.

Prana - Distinct from the subdosha of vata, prana in this sense means lifeforce.

Prana Vata - A subdosha of vata governing the inward movements of the body. For example, the intake of food or inhalation of air.

Pranayama - The conscious practice of controlling the breath. There are many forms of pranayama all with different effects.

Prashna - In the context of Ayurveda, prashna refers to the pulse reader's use of questioning to assist in the diagnosis of a rogi's condition.

Prithvi - Sanskrit word meaning "earth." In the context of Ayurveda the primary quality of prithvi is stability.

Pulse Reading - The art and science of perceiving and understanding patterns expressed by the pulse, communicating the status of the body.

R

Radial Artery - The primary site of pulse reading. It is located on the thumb's side of the wrist below the radial tubercle.

Rajas - One of the three mental gunas. Rajas initiates and sustains movement.

Rakta - One of the seven dhatus. Rakta is the constituent that forms blood.

Ranjaka Pitta - A subdosha of pitta located primarily in the liver. Ranjaka pitta gives color to blood, urine and feces.

Rasa - One of the seven dhatus. Rasa is the constituent of blood plasma. It carries nourishment to all of the other dhatus.

Rate - In the context of pulse reading, rate refers to how frequently the heart beats.

Rhythm - In the context of pulse reading, rhythm refers to the timing and regularity of pulse beats.

Rogi - One who is distressed. Or, one who is seeking the aid of a physician.

Root Cause - The primary causal factor in the pathology of a disease.

Often times, the root cause of a pathology is hidden. The root cause is not necessarily found at the location of manifesting symptoms. So long as the root cause is perpetuated, symptoms may subside but the pathology will not completely reverse and the rogi will remain out of balance.

S

Sadhaka Pitta - A subdosha of pitta located in the heart and brain. Sadhaka pitta governs discernment and intelligence.

Samana Vata - A subdosha of vata governing the linear movements of peristalsis through the gastrointestinal tract. It harmonizes the other subdoshas involved in digestion to ensure the proper breakdown of food.

Samprapti - The pathology of an imbalance. Samprapti has six distinct phases. Accumulation of the dosha in their seats, aggravation of the doshas within their seats, spread of the aggravated doshas from their seats, localization of the aggravated doshas in inappropriate dhatus and organs, manifestation of symptoms and differentiation of symptoms beginning a new, distinct pathology.

Sattva - One of the mental gunas. Sattva governs the appropriate use of rajas and tamas. It is clarity, neutrality, and balance.

Sheetali Pranayama - A specific breathing practice in which the practitioner curls his or her tongue into a "U" shape to inhale cool air into the body and then exhale through the nose. Sheetali pranayama is used to cool down the body and calm the mind.

Shleshaka Kapha - A subdosha of kapha located in the joints. It provides binding and lubrication within the joints.

Shukra Dhatu - One of the seven dhatus. Shukra is the constituent that forms reproductive tissue. It is found in every cell of the body and necessary for vitality.

Sparshana - In the context of Ayurveda, sparshana refers to the pulse reader's use of touch to assist in the diagnosis of a rogi's condition.

Subdosha - A particular functional aspect of one of the primary doshas.

Sunia - Deep listening from a calm and open heart and mind.

Sushumna - The central energetic channel running from the base of the spine to the top of the skull. A chakra is formed wherever it is crossed by the ida and pingala.

Sympathetic Nervous System - Part of the autonomic nervous system. The sympathetic nervous system governs heavy and quick actions. It is responsible for responding to threat and the defense mechanisms of fight, flight and freeze. While engaged, the body prioritizes the function of the peripheral limbs and the brain, and de-emphasizes digestive, restorative and reproductive functions.

T

Tamas - One of the three mental gunas. Tamas is inertia.
Tarpaka Kapha - One of the subdoshas of kapha located primarily in the cerebrospinal fluid, gray brain matter and white brain matter. It nourishes the entire nervous system.
Tejas - A highly refined form of pitta. Tejas is the focus and projection of attention.

U

Udana Vata - A subdosha of vata governing upward and outward movements such as exhalation.
Upadhatu - The upshot of a dhatu. Upadhatus are a particular form of their original dhatu to perform a specific function within the body.

V

Vagus Nerve - The tenth cranial nerve and the longest nerve in the body, innervating every vital organ. The vagus nerve relays information from the brain to the organs and from the organs to the brain. It governs the transition between the parasympathetic nervous system and the sympathetic nervous system.
Vata - One of the three primary doshas. Vata is composed of vayu and akash. It governs the all movements within the body, including the movement of information throughout the nervous system.
Vayu - Sanskrit word meaning "air." In the context of Ayurveda the primary quality of vayu is movement.
Vikruti - The state of imbalance in the context of an individual's prakruti.

Volume - In the context of pulse reading, volume refers to the amount of blood that travels through the veins and arteries at any given time.

Vyana Vata - A subdosha of vata governing centrifugal movements such as circulation from the heart to the extremities.

Y

Yoga - The union of individual consciousness with total consciousness.

REFERENCES

Babu, S. Suresh. *Yoga ratnākara: the "A" to "Z" Classic on Āyurvedic Formulations, Practices & Procedures, Sanskrit Text with English Translation and Explanatory Notes.* Vol. 1-2, Chowkhamba Sanskrit Series Office, 2005.

Bagwan Dash, R.K. Sharma, et al. *Charaka Samhita.* Vol. 1-7, Chaukhambha Publications, 2017.

Bloxham, Conor J, et al. "A Bitter Taste in Your Heart." *Frontiers in Physiology*, Frontiers Media S.A., 8 May 2020, www.ncbi. nlm.nih.gov/pmc/articles/PMC7225360/.

Frawley, David, and Suhas Kshirsagar. *The Art and Science of Vedic Counseling.* Motilal Banarsidass Publ, 2017.

Frawley, David. *Ayurveda and the Mind: the Healing of Consciousness.* Lotus, 2007.

Frawley, David. *Ayurvedic Healing: a Comprehensive Guide.* Motilal Banarsidass, 2003.

Gray, Henry F.R.S. *Gray's Anatomy.* Thunder Bay Press, 2001

Kaminoff, Leslie. *YOGA ANATOMY.* Calzetti E Mariucci, 2015.

Kshirsagar, Suhas G., et al. *Change Your Schedule, Change Your Life: How to Harness the Power of Clock Genes to Lose Weight, Optimize Your Workout, and Finally Get a Good Night's Sleep.* Harper Wave, an Imprint of HarperCollinsPublishers, 2019.

Kshirsagar, Suhas G., et al. *The Hot Belly Diet: a 30-Day Ayurvedic Plan to Reset Your Metabolism, Lose Weight, and Restore Your Body's Natural Balance to Heal Itself.* Atria Books, 2015.

Lad, Vasant. *Ayurveda: the Science of Self-Healing: a Practical Guide.* Lotus Press, 2009.

Lad, Vasant. *Secrets of the Pulse: the Ancient Art of Ayurvedic Pulse Diagnosis*. Ayurvedic Press, 2006.

Lele, Avinash, BAMS. Personal interview on ayurvedic herbology. 2 November, 2019.

Lele, Bharati, BAMS. Personal interview on ayurvedic nutrition. 30 October, 2019.

Lele, Nandan, BAMS. Personal interview series on ayurvedic anatomy and pathology. January - December, 2020.

Nanak, Guru. *Japji Sahib: the Song of the Soul*. Translated by Balkar Singh, Sikh Dharma International, 2004.

Pole, Sebastian. *Ayurvedic Medicine: the Principles of Traditional Practice*. Singing Dragon, 2013.

Porges, Stephen W. *The Polyvagal Theory*. W W Norton & Co Inc, 2017.

Rich, Joseph. Personal Interview on Horsemanship. 19 September, 2020

Rich, Joseph. Personal interview on the practices of Kundalini Yoga. 15, August 2020.

Singh Khalsa, Harbhajan. "Yogi Bhajan Lecture: The Power of the Third Chakra." *3HO*, 6 Apr. 2018, www.3ho.org/kundalini-yoga/chakras/yogi-bhajan-lecture-power-third-chakra.

Singhal, G. D. *Sushruta Samhita*. Vol. 1-3, Chowkhamba Sanskrit Series Office, 2018.

Soos, Michael P. "Sinus Arrhythmia." *StatPearls [Internet].*, U.S. National Library of Medicine, 24 Aug. 2020, www.ncbi.nlm.nih.gov/books/NBK537011/.

Teitelbaum, Marianne. *Healing the Thyroid with Ayurveda: Natural Treatments for Hashimoto's, Hypothyroidism, and Hyperthyroidism*. Healing Arts Press, 2019.

Vāgbhaṭa Vaidya. *Aṣṭāṅga hṛdaya Of Vāgbhaṭa*. Edited by Deepak Yadav, Chaukhambha Vishvabharati, 2016.

Vāgbhaṭa, Vaidya, and K. R. Srikanthamurthy. *Aṣṭāṅga Samgraha: Text, English Translation, Notes, Indeces, Etc.* Vol. 1-3, Chaukhambha Orientalia, 2005.

Vasav Rajiya Nadi Muhkta.

Vickery, Dia, DACM. Personal interview on styles of pulse reading in traditional Chinese Medicine. 29 September, 2020.

Wujastyk, Dominik. *The Roots of Ayurveda: Selectiond from Sanskrit Medical Writings*. Penguin Books, 2003.

Index

A

acharyas 28
agni (fire) 25
akash (ether) 25
  quality of, listening and 51
alochaka pitta 66
animals pulse 172
  dogs and cats 173
  horse 175
apana vata 64
  flow through kidneys 104
  function in liver 111
  in colon 106
  in gallbladder 109
asthi dhatu 81
avalambaka kapha 68, 70
  heart 96
  in lungs 108
  in pericardium 113
  in spleen 99
Ayurveda 1
  basics of 3
  solar and lunar channels in 37

B

bhrajaka pitta 66
bladder 102
bodhaka kapha 68
  small intestine 94
breathing, in pulse reading 12

C

cats pulse 173
  prakruti and vikruti, determining 175
  principles of reading 174
circulatory system 114
colon 105
communication 50
communication to rogi 138
  body language, paying attention to 143
  clarity 141

CONTINUE LEARNING WITH VICTOR

PULSE READING CASE STUDIES

Readers of this book have *free* access to the Pulse Reading Case Studies Website.

Visit www.pulseunveiled.com/login to create a private account.

The website hosts a compilation of anonymous client case studies from a number of different pulse readers. The website also includes other useful tools such as a pulse reading notation template.

CONTINUE YOUR TRAINING IN PERSON OR ONLINE

Victor offers both in person and online pulse reading training and workshops. Private sessions are also available.

Contact us at 707.225.8844 | victor@iitvsschool.org

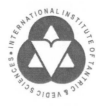

OTHER COURSES AT IITVS INCLUDE

Certified - Ayurvedic Practitioner Training
Taught by Victor Briere and Madison Madden
Certified - Panchakarma Technician Training
Taught by Madison Madden
Certified - Ayurveda, The Vagus Nerve and Addiction
Taught by Victor Briere

Contact us at 707.225.8844 | victor@iitvsschool.org

ABOUT VICTOR BRIERE

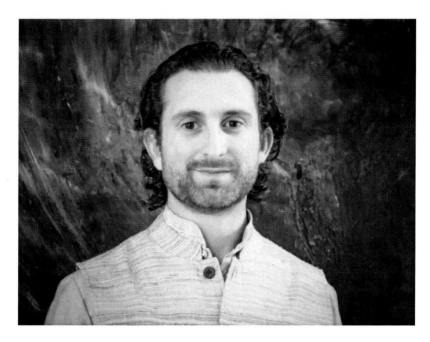

Victor is an Ayurvedic Doctor and co-founder of, Pacific Coast Ayurveda. It is in the clinic where he applies his knowledge of pulse reading daily. The clinic is an active place of healing for all those who seek a semblance of balance and health in the modern world.

Victor is also the co-founder and faculty of The International Institute of Tantric and Vedic Sciences (IITVS). IITVS is an ayurvedic school that trains and certifies ayurvedic practitioners, pulse readers, panchakarma technicians, and hosts a number of ayurvedic and yogic workshops each year.

Victor learned the art of pulse reading from Dr. Suhas Kshirsagar, Dr. Vasant Lad, and has worked directly with thousands of clients. He is forever a student of the pulse, continuously searching for timeless pulse reading wisdom both within the clinic and from seasoned pulse readers around the world.

ABOUT VICTOR'S COMMUNITY

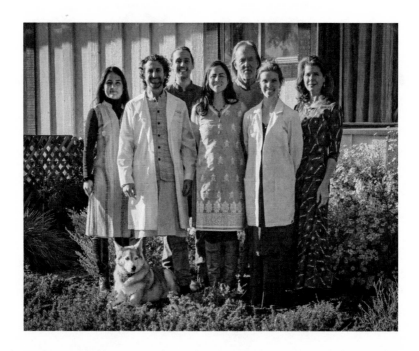

There is no real way to get to know Victor without also getting to know his community. They are a group of vibrant yogis and yoginis living an ayurvedic life in Northern California. Victor is a co-founder of Pacific Coast Ayurveda, an ayurvedic clinic and panchakarma center, alongside Madison Madden, AD. The Guru's Kitchen, an ayurvedic, vegetarian kitchen and bakery serving the community at large is an essential element of Pacific Coast Ayurveda.

The kitchen is run by Gurubhai, the yoga teacher for the community and co-founder of Pacific Coast Ayurveda. Patrick focuses on applying the wisdom of yoga and ayurveda to shifting attitudes towards environmental consciousness while conveniently working as close to the bakery as possible. Lisa supports the community through her wide range of professional connections and with her "producer's eye" on all community happenings. Oceanne is a panchakarma therapist in the clinic and a cook in the kitchen. Jennifer, Victor's wife, operates the business side of all the community's operations.